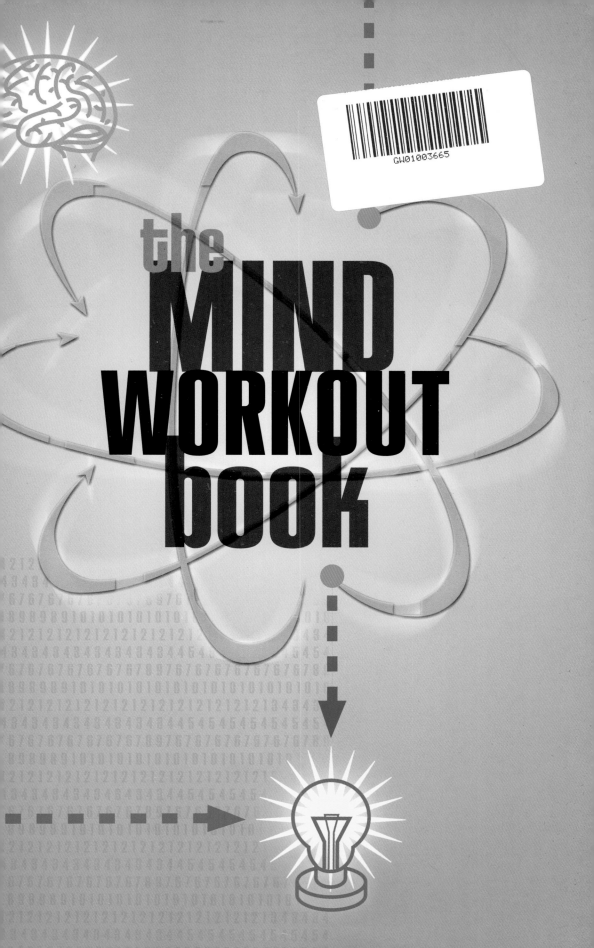

the **MIND WORKOUT book**

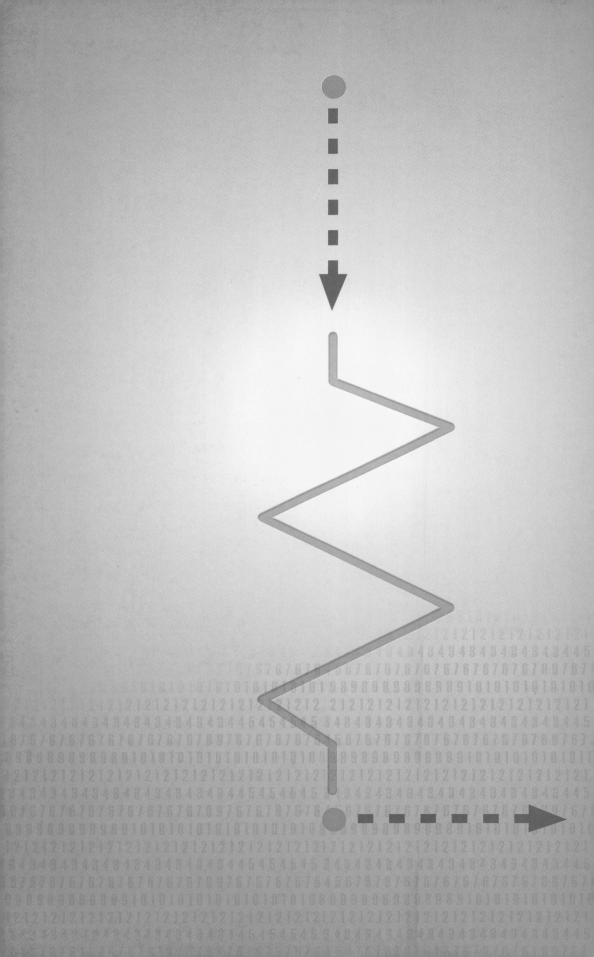

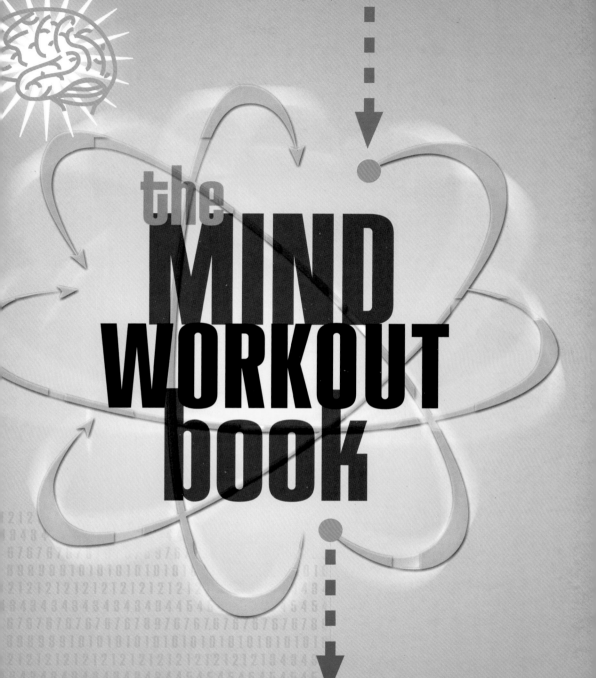

the MIND WORKOUT book

ROBERT ALLEN

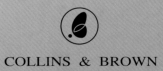

COLLINS & BROWN

First published in Great Britain in 2003 by
Collins & Brown Ltd
The Chrysalis Building
Bramley Road
London W10 6SP

An imprint of **Chrysalis** Books Group plc

Project Manager: Nicola Hodgson
Editor: Constance Novis
Designer: Zoë Mellors
Illustrator: Jon Morgan

10 9 8 7 6 5 4 3 2

British Library Cataloguing-in-Publication Data:
A catalogue record for this title is available from the British Library.

ISBN 1–84340–101–0 (hb)

Reproduced by Classicscan Pte Ltd
Printed by SNP Leefung Printers Ltd,China

Contents

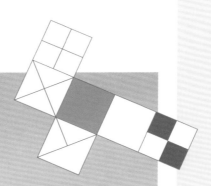

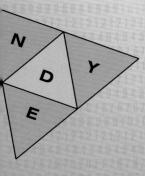

Introduction

When you think about it, your mind is all you've got. Everything that makes up your life is actually a function of your mind. Even your body is only available to you as a mind object. Anything that is outside your mind simply does not exist. You can't even think about it because, if you could, it would then immediately be inside your mind. It is therefore strange that we take the mind so much for granted. We spend our childhood and maybe even our early adult years having information (much of it utterly useless) pumped into us whether we like it or not and then ... nothing. After formal teaching ceases, the mind is left to get with it and is largely ignored for the rest of our lives. What a tragedy! Imagine having such a splendid instrument at your disposal and not doing as much with it as you could!

This book seeks to correct this situation. It provides you with exercises that will enhance your mind power in a number of highly important areas. One of the most basic is what we have called Mind Development. Because we have not been taught how to use our minds they remain undeveloped. Our society has no tradition of mind development so we have never been given the tools necessary to do it. Fortunately for us, other civilizations have developed such tools, such as meditation, and these are now available to us. Even though it has been talked of here since the '60s, meditation is still widely misunderstood and confused in the popular mind with 'Eastern mysticism', whatever that is supposed to mean. In fact meditation is not one thing but a whole variety of mind-training methods that can bring huge advantages to those who choose to practise them.

Also included in the book are exercises in concentration. Think back to your school days and to the number of times teachers told you to concentrate. But did they even teach you how? Concentration is not something that just happens, it has to be learned and practised until it becomes as natural to you as breathing. The same goes for memory. A certain type of old-fashioned teacher was always very keen on you learning material by heart, but did they ever teach you how? Of course not. Yet memory is just like a muscle – the more you use it, the stronger it gets. And not only that, there are tricks that will make your memory even stronger. In fact it is possible to fix some information so firmly in your memory that you will retain it for life. This book will teach you how to do that.

This book also teaches you about creativity. If you've never thought of yourself as a particularly creative person then it's time all that changed. The first and most important step to being creative is to make a once-and-for-all decision that says, 'Yes, I am a creative person.' From then on your thoughts are not longer random mental doodling but become valuable ideas that may, with a bit of work, be transformed into something startlingly new and useful. How do you get creative ideas? The problem is that no one really knows. They are thrown up by the subconscious pretty much at random. However, everybody is capable of having them, you just have to give them a bit of encouragement. Remember the story of how Benjamin Franklin flew kites with a key attached in order to encourage lightning to strike so he could study electricity? Well, creativity is a bit like that – you have to encourage a sort of mental lightning to strike. The exercises in this book will not only help lightning to strike but will also help you to recognize good ideas when they arrive.

The book also focuses on helping you get to grips with problem solving. This is another facet of your mental life you probably haven't looked at since school. It was unpleasant to sit in a stuffy classroom being made to think logically. But now that you don't have to do it, you'll find it can be both pleasurable and useful. After all, if you don't manage to get the right answer, you won't have to stay behind after school, will you? Some people have been so traumatized by nasty school experiences that they now say things like, 'I don't mind solving real world problems but I don't see the point of sitting around wasting time on puzzles.' This translates as, 'I'm not sure that I can do this and I don't want to look a fool.' Don't worry! You will be able to do it and, with a bit of effort, you'll get better and better at it. The sort of thinking you need to solve puzzles is useful in real life and it's a pity that it has such a bad reputation. Give it a try and you won't be disappointed.

Lateral thinking is another area investigated in the book. Since the '70s lateral thinking has been popular but mainly as a sort of party game. There is, however, a lot more to it than that. Once you get used to the idea of not letting your thinking processes plod along in a straight line you'll also find that all sorts of different and interesting solutions become available to you. This book provides you with a number of problems to practise on but, when you've finished these, it would be a good idea to try to incorporate this method into your normal problem-solving toolkit.

14 7 3 7 3 5 4 6 2 8 5 4

The book has been compiled with the idea that the tasks should be fun rather than 'good for you'. It will limber you up mentally, awaken abilities you didn't know you had and improve on faculties that may have got a bit rusty over the years. You do not have to tackle the whole thing at once, you can do as much or as little as you please, you can spend a lot of time on activities that please you and a little (or none at all) on those that you don't like.

36 4 4 5 7 3 7 2 8 2 3 7

53 7 5 2 4 6 7 2 2 8 7 3

84 6 4 3 7 5 5 7 3 6 2 8

90 4 6 3 5 5 1 9 4 5 2 8

You will almost certainly find that the tasks will spark off new interests and that you will rush off full of enthusiasm to pursue interests that you had not thought of before. 'Your book's a bit like manure really,' a friend told me. 'What do you mean?' I asked, not entirely sure that I was keen on the tone of this conversation. 'Well, it helps people grow, doesn't it?' Ah, yes, good point. That's exactly what it does.

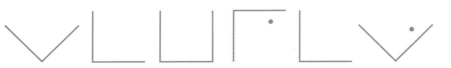

How to use this book

There are over 100 questions throughout the workout directory section. You can either work through them all sequentially or use the cross-references beneath each task that take you on a less linear route. Each task appears with its category symbol and is graded for level of difficulty: simple, moderate or hard, helping you to pick out questions that are relevant to your own needs.

Be sure to work on the Mind Development tasks at a pace that suits you. All the techniques are completely safe but, unlike physical exercise, where the ache of tired muscles warns you to take a rest, unfamiliar mental exertion can exhaust you without you realizing. Just work at a modest pace and build up stamina as you go along. These exercises are enormously beneficial and, practised regularly over a long period, will have a dramatic effect on your wellbeing and that of those around you.

Look at the following questions. If you answer YES to more than five of them then this is a category you should pay attention to as you work through the book.

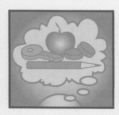

MEMORY
Memory is like a muscle; the more you use it the stronger it gets. Illness and stress may briefly affect it but if you make a habit of memorizing, you'll retain a reliable memory.

Questions
1. Do you fail to put names to faces?
2. Do you forget appointments?
3. Do you get embarrassed about introducing people in case you forget their name?
4. Do you forget where you put stuff?
5. Is it hard to memorize facts and figures?
6. Have you entered a room and forgotten why?
7. Do you forget where you parked your car or bike?
8. Do you forget birthdays and anniversaries?
9. Do you get lost easily?
10. Do you forget tasks you intended to complete?

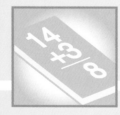

PROBLEM SOLVING
If you find it hard to think your way out of a brown paper bag, this is the section for you. It will help your logical powers become razor-sharp.

Questions
1. Do you struggle with IQ questions?
2. Do you avoid problem solving or making decisions?
3. Do you draw up lists before you make a decision?
4. Does logic make your brain ache?
5. Would you rather leave someone else to do the hard thinking?
6. Would you like to solve problems more efficiently?
7. Do you find your colleagues are often quicker at coming up with the right answer?
8. Are you ashamed by the slowness of your mental processes?
9. Do you struggle with figures?
10. Do you find crosswords simply beyond you?

COMMUNICATION

Effective contact is essential to all successful relations. Sometimes we use words, but most of the messages we send are non-verbal. This section will build both verbal and non-verbal communication skills.

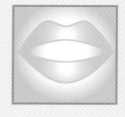

Questions

1. Do you ever feel you give people mixed signals?
2. Do you often struggle to find the right word?
3. Ever find it hard to express yourself?
4. Do people ever misunderstand you?
5. Do you hate 'just-passing-the-day' conversations?
6. Do you express simple views in a long-winded way?
7. Are you aware of the effect you have on others?
8. Is it ever hard for you to put across your point of view?
9. Do you feel disadvantaged in an argument?
10. Is it ever difficult to reach a word that's just on the tip of your tongue?

CREATIVITY

Creativity is highly valued but rarely taught. The creativity tasks will give an extra sparkle to everything you do and make your efforts stand out from the crowd.

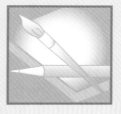

Questions

1. Do you feel you sometimes lack imagination?
2. Would you like to express yourself in a more spontaneous style in written correspondence?
3. Do you find 'colouring in' therapeutic?
4. Does your work give you little scope to express your personality?
5. Do you find it hard to come up with bright ideas?
6. Do you fall back on accepted ways of doing things rather than think of a new one?
7. Do you find your thinking is often a little conventional?
8. When you redecorate do you find yourself reusing the same old colour schemes that you had before?
9. Is your personal image getting a bit stale?
10. Do you think people find you just a bit too predictable?

MIND DEVELOPMENT

This section deals with deep relaxation, concentration and visualization. It will help you revitalize and improve some important existing mental powers and discover others you perhaps didn't know you possessed.

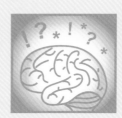

Questions

1. Do you find it hard to unwind at the end of the day?
2. Do you regularly suffer from insomnia?
3. Do you take your worries from work to bed with you?
4. Are you easily distracted from tasks?
5. Do you find it hard to work for long periods without a break?
6. Do you find it hard to take in complex information?
7. Do you find it hard to play games demanding concentration, such as bridge or chess?
8. Do you find that your mind wanders if you drive for a long time?
9. Do you have trouble visualizing situations and outcomes?
10. Do you have poor visual imagination?

KEY

Task category

5 seconds

10 minutes

1 hour

unlimited time

MODERATE
Level of difficulty

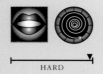

HARD

1 Backwards

AIM Here's a communication game with a difference. You'll probably prefer to play this with people you know well, though. For those who are uninhibited, it makes a great introduction.

TASK For this game you need some adverbs written on slips of paper. Words such as aggressively, playfully, strongly, gently, lovingly, etc., will be fine. One player picks up a slip and reads it but keeps the contents secret. Two players then stand back to back and the one who has read the adverb tries to express it solely by rubbing backs with the partner. This game can be a serious exercise in communication (which is, of course, the only reason it has been included), but at the right sort of party it can also be a lot of fun.

POOR	AVERAGE	BRILLIANT
Couldn't do it? Try again and this time change the rules so that you get to choose the word you express. Try ➤ Task 17	If you had some success with this one keep trying and put in some harder words. Try 'enigmatically'! Try ➤ Task 29	If you were good at this try ➤ Task 34

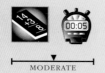

MODERATE

2 Parts Problem

AIM There is no time in this test to use any reasoning powers, so you must rely solely on the acuity of your visual judgment.

TASK All you have to do is glance at the diagrams right for only five seconds and then decide which two figures contain the greatest number of segments.

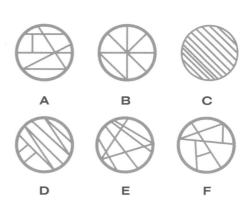

A   B   C

D   E   F

POOR	AVERAGE	BRILLIANT
If you were fooled into choosing D that's because it was made to look more complex than it is. Try ➤ Task 15	If you got at least one of the figures right in the time allowed, that's not bad. Try ➤ Task 19	If you saw through this problem literally at a glance your visual judgement is excellent. Try ➤ Task 33

3 Basic Meditation

HARD

AIM Contrary to Western belief, the term meditation covers a huge variety of quite different techniques. This is a beginner's technique that will help you access other forms of meditation. Don't make the mistake of dismissing meditation as useless 'navel gazing'. It is a very powerful method of self-development and is suitable for just about anybody. As taught in this book it has no religious connotations and will not come into conflict with whatever beliefs you may hold.

TASK Sit on an upright chair but don't lean against the back. Sit up straight but don't strain. You should feel comfortable. Fold your hands in your lap and close your eyes. Now start to count your breaths. Count 'one' as you breathe in, 'two' as you breathe out. Keep going until you arrive at 'ten'. Then start again. Don't attempt to breathe deeply. This may sound easy but your mind will wander constantly and you'll probably lose count. Don't worry, every time you discover your mind wandering, just gently bring it back and focus once again on your breathing. Keep this up for 15 minutes and repeat daily.

POOR	AVERAGE	BRILLIANT
Couldn't concentrate? Kept thinking of things you should be doing? Try shortening the time you take. It's far better to do five minutes properly than 15 badly. But don't give up because those who find it most difficult often get great benefits when they learn to do this well. Try ❱❱ Task 11	If you managed to get through the 15 minutes then keep on practising. You will find that it takes time to make real progress. Don't be in any hurry to move on. Wait until you are really at ease and find that the 15 minutes feels like a pleasurable eternity. Try ❱❱ Task 18	Those who manage the beginners' exercise easily can try ❱❱ Task 37

Doing the task 'I sat there feeling bored and itchy. Nothing happened.' If that's your reaction you are not unusual. Did you ever learn a language? How much did you understand after the first lesson? Exactly. Meditation takes time and effort to do well. It is not like anything you've learnt before and, if you want to succeed, you need to persist with it.

HELP
When you sit down to meditate do it as though you never intend to get up again. Give up everyday thoughts completely and focus your whole mind on what you are doing.

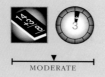

MODERATE

4 Misfit

AIM Recognizing categories is an important mental ability. When we see something new for the first time we perform an instant sorting programme that tells us whether we can eat it, write with it or put it on the wall as a decoration, etc. Because we have a huge library of categories built up over years of experience, the process is usually instantaneous and we are not even aware of it. But what happens when you don't know what categories to use? Try this puzzle and find out.

TASK These words may appear to be quite unrelated but they have something in common. When you work out what it is you will be able to spot the one that doesn't fit.

APRIL   HOLLY   CHARITY   DANDELION   SANDY   INDIA

POOR	**AVERAGE**	**BRILLIANT**
Try something new.	Got it after a bit of thought? OK.	No problems here?
➤ Task 9	Try ➤ Task 15	Try ➤ Task 28

DOING THE TASK Ask yourself, is this about the words themselves, about the letters that compose the words or is there something else?

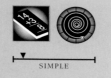

SIMPLE

5 Bullets

AIM This is an exercise to help you get to the nub of communication.

TASK Take a piece of writing such as a newspaper or magazine article and read it carefully. Now simply reduce the whole thing to a series of bullet points. It is surprising how much verbiage journalists, supposedly skilled writers, include just for decoration. Of course, a story that consisted of nothing but bullet points wouldn't be very interesting to read, but at least you would know all the important facts. This is a really important exercise that many people never do. If you fail to analyze information in this way you can come away with a completely false impression. For example, an article with the headline, 'Redheads should be banned from public places', could be sinister and disturbing if it were to turn out to be government policy but merely silly and provocative if it emanated from the Blonde Protection League.

HELP
If you have difficulty picking out the facts just ask yourself: Where? When? Who? Why? How? Which? You will also find that 'How much?' comes into most stories.

POOR	**AVERAGE**	**BRILLIANT**
This might require a bit of practice but it is an important skill to acquire.	Try ➤ Task 20	Try ➤ Task 32
Try ➤ Task 16		

6 Random Stanzas

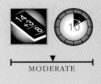

SIMPLE

AIM This is another exercise that will allow you to get past that creative block and reach the fertile soil of your unconscious mind.

TASK Take some small slips of paper and write one of your favourite words on one side of each one. Favourite words? That's right, just choose words that you really like the sound of. You need at least 100 words but the more the better. When you've got all your words ready, turn the slips of paper face down on the table and give them a good stir so that you have no idea which is which. Then start to pick words at random. Pick as many as you like and then, when you decide you have enough, start to move them around to form sentences. Of course, you won't get complete grammatical sentences without much use of your imagination, but you will get phrases that suggest ideas to you. How you use these phrases is up to you. You could write a poem, produce the first line of a story or find a key phrase that will help you solve a problem.

POOR
If words don't hold much attraction for you, then this technique may not work too well. Try something more visual ➤ Task 50

AVERAGE
If you have some success with this, keep developing your collection of words. The bigger your special vocabulary is, the more ideas it can express. Try ➤ Task 59

BRILLIANT
If this really helps you, then make sure that you enlarge your vocabulary regularly and always consult it when trying to find a new idea. Try ➤ Task 70

7 Boudicca's Birthday

MODERATE

AIM Here's a problem that will test your mathematical skills.

TASK Boudicca died 129 years after Cleopatra was born. If you add their ages at death together you get 100. Cleopatra died in 30 BC. So when was Boudicca born?

POOR
If you can't do this one you need to get your head round the fact that there is a gap between the two lives and there is a simpler way of working out what that gap is. When you've got it try ➤ Task 35

AVERAGE
This is one of those puzzles that are 'easy when you know how it's done'. If you worked it out, well done. Try ➤ Task 48

BRILLIANT
If this is all like mother's milk to you then clearly maths is your forte. Try ➤ Task 51

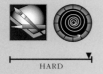

HARD

8 Dots and Splashes

AIM This is a tricky task that had its origins in the paintings of ancient China. It may seem easy at first but it is actually very hard. It works on a strange principle that induces you to be creative by forcing you to be deliberately as uncreative as possible. Intrigued? Read on.

TASK Take a sheet of paper, some black ink and a brush. Now begin to place dots and splashes on the paper. This, however, is not some sort of Rorschach Blot Test in which you are invited to see patterns in random marks. In this case there is a strict rule that you must not make any patterns. Easy? Go ahead and try! The more you struggle not to create patterns, the more they will insist on emerging. The chances are that you will eventually produce something that has creative potential.

> It's hard to fail at this exercise. Either you succeed in producing a non-pattern, which is what you were asked to do, or your creative powers take over and produce something beautiful in spite of your efforts to restrain them. Try ❯❯ Task 20

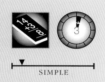

SIMPLE

9 Letter Logic 1

AIM This task tests vocabulary. It shouldn't strain the grey matter to breaking point but you might need to nibble the end of your pencil lightly.

TASK Take the second letter in each pair of the words below and change it for another letter to make two new words. For example, STUMP ( ) CROCK would give L (SLUMP and CLOCK). If you write the new letters in the central brackets you will find that they spell a word.

ABSENT	( )	ALTER
STAMP	( )	ONE
NONE	( )	CONCH
SPILE	( )	OPEN
ERE	( )	EVER
BIND	( )	POKE
WITCH	( )	SLID
COOP	( )	FLOG

POOR	AVERAGE	BRILLIANT
Keep trying.	You got this within	Try something
Try ❯❯ Task 28	the time?	more challenging.
	Try ❯❯ Task 36	Try ❯❯ Task 35

10 Hanky Habit

MODERATE

AIM Have you ever reminded yourself to do something by tying a knot in your handkerchief? It may be a bit childish (you probably used it to remind you to take your bus money to school) but it works.

TASK Devise a number of other physical tricks to assist your memory. You can leave things out of their normal places in your home or office or perhaps put some unusual object on your desk.

POOR	**AVERAGE**	**BRILLIANT**
Try ➤ Task 13	Try ➤ Task 14	Try ➤ Task 22

11 Basic Visualization

SIMPLE

AIM Visualization is simply a technique whereby you create mental pictures. By doing this you can alter your mood in a number of important ways. First, you will learn to create calm, happy moods that will increase your inner peace. Second, by imagining how you will deal with a difficult situation, you can prepare yourself to handle it better. More controversially, many people believe that by visualizing a desired outcome, they can bring it about in reality.

TASK Some people have great visual imagination, while others have little or none. Here's a very easy exercise for those who are not quite sure which category they fall into. You should sit comfortably, close your eyes and imagine in as much detail as possible how you would carry out a very simple task like, for example, making a sandwich. Work at capturing every detail in your mind's eye. Get the bread out of the bread bin, look at its colour and texture, fetch the butter and sandwich filling from the fridge. Take a knife out and carefully spread the butter and then the filling. Place the top slice on the sandwich and cut the whole thing in half. Then picture yourself washing the knife and putting it back in the drawer. Did you make yourself feel so hungry that you needed a real sandwich afterwards? Success!

POOR	**AVERAGE**	**BRILLIANT**
If you can't do this at all, then it's possible that visualization is not for you. Before you give up, go back and have another go at **Candle Power** ➤ Task 109.	If you managed this one well enough, go and try ➤ Task 21	If you found this very easy, then pass on quickly to ➤ Task 25

HELP
The success of visualization is in the detail. It is necessary to observe the things you want to visualize very closely (just as you would if you wanted to draw them) and then file away mental pictures of what they look like.

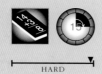

12 Dear Departed

AIM This is a rather tricky logic puzzle based on an actual epitaph dating from 1538. See if you can work out the relationships involved.

TASK

Two grandmothers with their two granddaughters,

Two husbands with their two wives,

Two fathers with their two daughters,

Two mothers with their two sons,

Two maidens with their two mothers,

Two sisters with their two brothers,

Yet only six lie buried here,

All born legitimate, from incest clear.

POOR	AVERAGE	BRILLIANT
Didn't get it?	Congratulations!	If you found this easy
Try ≫ Task 19	Try ≫ Task 22	Try ≫ Task 28

HELP
It is not obvious but the puzzle involves in-laws.

Doing the task Like most apparently complex relationship problems, the answer is really very simple but rather unlikely.

13 Ritual

AIM A memory ritual is a set of actions, the more bizarre the better, designed to remind you of something important you must do.

TASK My elder cousin used to remind herself to wake up at a certain time by programming her body clock with a ritual. As she went to bed she'd turn around three times while tapping herself three times on the head at each turn and repeating out loud the time at which she wanted to wake. (See task 125 to see how you can also use the body clock itself as a reminder.) Your task is to construct a ritual that will remind you of some important event of your choice. In order to work efficiently the ritual should be strange enough to embed itself in your unconscious and prompt your memory at the appropriate time.

HELP
Why go to all this trouble when you could set an alarm clock? Well, memory is like a muscle, the more you use it the stronger it gets. By relying on machines or written notes we weaken our power to remember. If you make a habit of giving your memory a workout it will continue to look after you even when you get older.

POOR	AVERAGE	BRILLIANT
Perhaps the ritual was just a bit too restrained.	If this worked up to a point, keep practising and improve your skills.	This one really worked for you? Excellent!
Try ≫ Task 14	Try ≫ Task 27	Try ≫ Task 31

14 Kim's Game 1

AIM This is a simple memory game that you probably played at parties. Nevertheless it is a good way to limber up those memory muscles in preparation for the harder tasks ahead.

TASK Look at the illustration for two minutes and try to memorize all of the items. Then close the book and write a list of everything you saw.

SIMPLE

POOR
If you managed to recall fewer than half of the objects your memory muscles need some hard exercise.
➤ Task **27**

AVERAGE
If you managed to remember at least nine of the objects, go straight to Kim's Game 2
➤ Task **42**

BRILLIANT
If you remembered all of the objects, go to Kim's Game 3 ➤ Task **87**

HELP
With this exercise it's better to take a mental snapshot of the objects rather than trying to learn them as a list. Close your eyes and visualize all the objects just as they are in our illustration.

MODERATE

15 Triangle Trouble

AIM This is another logical challenge that hinges on the question, 'How does it work?' Once you see a pattern you should have no trouble getting to the answer.

TASK Look at the triangles and work out which letter should replace the question mark.

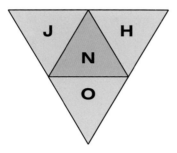

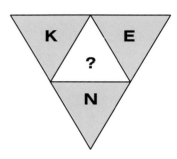

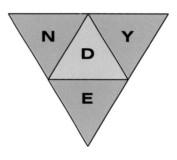

POOR
If you didn't get this you maybe need to be a bit more flexible in your thinking.
Try ❯❯ Task 45

AVERAGE
If you worked it out after a struggle you can try ❯❯ Task 50

BRILLIANT
If this struck you as really easy, try ❯❯ Task 56

HELP
Don't let yourself be fooled into looking for complexities. Often answers are obvious if you just know the right way to look at the problem.

Doing the task Older readers have a better chance with this one than youngsters. Even so it shouldn't present an insuperable problem. Look at the top left triangle first and see if it gives you any ideas.

16 You're just Putty in my Hands

AIM This is a creativity game that will probably appeal more to youngsters, though adults can play it if they are sufficiently uninhibited. It allows two people at a time to exercise different creative abilities.

TASK All the players form a circle and one is chosen to start. The aim is to make something recognizable (a rabbit, for example) from a blob of imaginary modelling clay. The person on your left has to work out what you are making. When they get it right you hand them the clay and they get to roll it up into a ball and make something of their own. Speaking or any sort of noise made by the person doing the model is cheating.

SIMPLE

POOR
If you find the models hard to make, try keeping to simple shapes. When guessing look at the basic shape first, then the details.
Try ⇥ Task 20

AVERAGE
If you have some success at this you can try it with more ambitious models.
Try ⇥ Task 24

BRILLIANT
Try ⇥ Task 32

HELP
Keep it simple until you've developed some skill at this game. Trying to make a vase of flowers at this early stage is just going to confuse everyone.

17 Tent Tantrums

AIM This is a communication exercise that will drive everybody mad. But it does highlight real problems and gets you to think about how best to deal with them.

HARD

TASK The classic form of this game calls for a small tent though, in practice, you could substitute all sorts of other objects that will need to be constructed from a variety of parts. One player is the leader and has to instruct the others in how to put the tent together. Easy so far? Yes, but the twist is that the workers are all blindfolded. Success depends on the leader being concise and accurate when giving instructions, and the workers following orders intelligently. You will either end up with a harmonious exercise in communication and a nicely erected tent, or civil war and a heap of plastic.

POOR
You aren't on speaking terms and the tent lies in a tangle on the floor? Oops!
Try ⇥ Task 26

AVERAGE
If you got the tent up, why not try again and, this time, allow yourselves less time.
Try ⇥ Task 34

BRILLIANT
Keep doing this, changing your leader at each new attempt, and see what your best time is.
Try ⇥ Task 46

HELP
The leader needs to be articulate, concise and well organized. The workers should follow instructions and not try to take over the process.

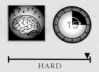

HARD

18 Mandala Meditation

AIM A mandala is a design that represents the universe. For those with a good visual imagination they make excellent objects for meditation. If you have completed some of the visualization exercises in this book and feel confident of your abilities, then see how you make out with the mandala shown below.

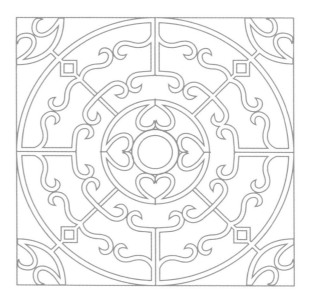

TASK The mandala above is a simple one for practice purposes. Once you get proficient at this form of meditation there are thousands of other more complicated and colourful examples available in books or on the internet. Follow the procedure described in Candle Power on page 95 but this time, instead of concentrating on a candle, use the mandala above. It is quite complicated so it will take some time and effort to call it to mind. Once you have the shape of the mandala fixed firmly in your mind you will find that, as you meditate on it, it begins to glow. Even though this pattern is monochrome it will take on colours of its own and the more you use it the more spectacular it will become. Certain mandalas are reputed to have special powers and a little research will help you find one that is exactly suited to your needs.

HELP
Start from the centre of the pattern and, when you have got that fixed in your mind, move outwards adding extra details as you go.

POOR
If you can't make this work for you then go to
➤ Task 11

AVERAGE
If you find that you can do this but only with difficulty, either persist until the task becomes easier or change to one of the breathing methods in
➤ Task 54

BRILLIANT
If you have strong visual abilities and this method really works for you then you could also try the visual memory techniques in
➤ Task 43

19 Princess Yasmin's Maze

AIM This is a simple test of your non-verbal reasoning skills. It involves a certain amount of logic but the main emphasis is on your ability to process visual information quickly. Five seconds may not seem long for this puzzle but there is a very obvious way to find the answer.

SIMPLE

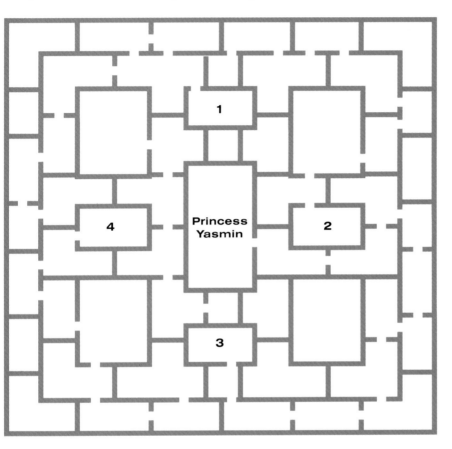

TASK Princess Yasmin's father insists that she get married. There are four princes competing for her hand. She convinces her dad that they should be put to a test. Each suitor has one hour to find his way to Yasmin's private chamber. The man who arrives first gets the bride. Yasmin, who has already seen the suitors and knows which one she wants, has rigged the game. Little do they know that only one of them has any chance of completing the task. Which suitor is it?

POOR	AVERAGE	BRILLIANT
You took ages to find the path? Never mind. Try a different sort of visual puzzle. Try ➤ Task 33	If you got the answer in about five seconds, try the maze in ➤ Task 78	Well done! Test your problem-solving skills further with ➤ Task 44

Doing the task It's easiest to start from the end and work backwards.

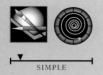

SIMPLE

20 Think Creative

AIM The only way to be creative is to believe that you are creative. This task gives you a push in the right direction.

TASK If you want to increase your creativity you have to work at it day and night. Your first task is simply to convince yourself that you are a creative person. From now on your thoughts, experiences, dreams, doodles and even the things you overhear other people say, will all be grist to your mill. Collect everything. Throw nothing away. All of it, sooner or later, will prove useful. Here are just a few of the things you can do to enhance your creativity:

- Keep a diary or, at the very least, a notebook of your ideas.

- Pay close attention to dreams. They are often a good source of inspiration.

- If you doodle during idle moments, hang on to your doodles.

- Make a point of having new experiences that give you a chance to broaden your mind.

- Listen not just to what people say, but the way that they say it. Casual remarks made by other people can be an excellent trigger for bright ideas.

- Never question whether you have a creative gift (plenty of other people will do that for you). Just keep on creating and, eventually, someone will spot your potential.

- Always pay attention to other people's best ideas, not to copy them but because one good idea can often spark off another.

POOR
If you don't do any of the things outlined above you'll find that being creative is almost impossible. If you get nothing else from this section you should pay attention to this page.
Try ⇒ Task 29

AVERAGE
The more you think of yourself as creative the more creative you will become. Hold on to all your ideas. Even apparently bad ideas are worth keeping on record as they sometimes turn out to be good ideas in disguise.
Try ⇒ Task 41

BRILLIANT
If this all comes naturally to you so much the better.
Try ⇒ Task 59

21 Picking Pairs

AIM This is a way to build your concentration. It looks really simple but unless you remain completely focused you will not do very well.

TASK Take a look at the rows of figures below. In each row you must pick out pairs of adjacent numbers that add up to 10. For example, in this line: 3 4 6 5 2 8 9 3 7, there are three pairs (4 + 6, 2 + 8 and 3 + 7). If you had a line containing 4 6 4 that would count as TWO pairs.

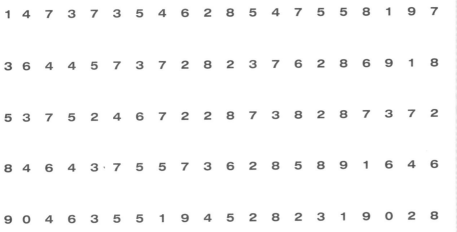

1 4 7 3 7 3 5 4 6 2 8 5 4 7 5 5 8 1 9 7

3 6 4 4 5 7 3 7 2 8 2 3 7 6 2 8 6 9 1 8

5 3 7 5 2 4 6 7 2 2 8 7 3 8 2 8 7 3 7 2

8 4 6 4 3 · 7 5 5 7 3 6 2 8 5 8 9 1 6 4 6

9 0 4 6 3 5 5 1 9 4 5 2 8 2 3 1 9 0 2 8

POOR	AVERAGE	BRILLIANT
If you found fewer than 25 pairs your concentration is poor. Do the exercise again and see if you can improve your score. Have another go at Candle Power in » Task 109. Then go forward to Alphabet Soup in » Task 98	If you found 28–34 pairs, that's not bad at all though there is room for improvement. There is no point repeating this exercise but you should have another go at Candle Power in » Task 109 before trying Alphabet Soup in » Task 98	If you found 35–39 pairs your concentration is excellent. You might not want to bother with Alphabet Soup in » Task 98 but could go straight to Sarah's Game in » Task 25

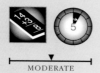

MODERATE

22 Sentence Search

AIM Here's a verbal reasoning test. It's not that difficult once you make a breakthrough but it has the capacity to confuse.

TASK The grid contains a short sentence. To find it you must follow the letters from square to touching square in any direction.

	T	I	S	
A	R	M	O	N
I	P	S	T	H
O	I	E	O	G
	T	N	U	

POOR
If you are having trouble, the knack is to look for the small words first and see if they lead you to the longer ones. You can see ARM, SIT, NOT, IS and others. Look at what surrounds them and see whether you are on the right track. When you are finished try ➨ Task 40

AVERAGE
The sentence, though not in any way difficult, is not the type that you say every day. Was it enough to put you off? No? Damn!
Try ➨ Task 82

BRILLIANT
If you saw through this within seconds you obviously have a gift for verbal reasoning. Time for something different.
Try ➨ Task 16

23 Ball Bother

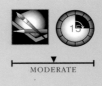

MODERATE

AIM To be successful at lateral thinking you must consider all the possibilities. Instead of 'lateral' thinking it should have been called flexible thinking. Lateral thinking doesn't use any different type of logic. It just depends on the exploration of unusual avenues. The following puzzle works on the assumption that you will instinctively shy away from the correct line of enquiry.

TASK Two small brothers are playing with a ping-pong ball when, to their dismay, it falls down a hole that is only just larger than the ball. There is no way they can get their fingers or any other implement into the hole to pull the ball out. They can't leave their playroom or their mother will realize something is wrong. They are afraid to call for help because they think they'll get told off. How do they get the ball out of the hole?

POOR
If you didn't get this one you might be insufficiently flexible or just too squeamish. Try ⯮ Task 91

AVERAGE
If you got it, then well done. Try ⯮ Task 85

BRILLIANT
If you got this one after only a moment's thought, well done! Try ⯮ Task 36

24 Psychiatrist

MODERATE

AIM This is an excellent game for solving problems creatively. You need quite a large group of people who know each other to make it work properly – a school or office group would be ideal.

TASK Six people volunteer to be patients and form a circle. One of the non-patients either volunteers or is chosen to be the psychiatrist and then takes a position in the centre of the circle. The object of the game is for the psychiatrist to work out what is wrong with the patients by asking them questions about themselves. When he or she has an answer it may be whispered to one of the patients. If it is the right answer then the psychiatrist joins the circle of patients and another non-player joins in as psychiatrist. The secret is that each patient thinks that he or she is the person to his or her left and answers all questions as that person. Though the secret is simple it takes quite a creative leap to work it out.

POOR
Try asking some very personal questions to which you already know the answer. Try ⯮ Task 19

AVERAGE
The more personal your questions, the better your chances of cracking it. Try ⯮ Task 27

BRILLIANT
Got is straight away? Well done! Try ⯮ Task 125

HELP
The answer is staring you in the face. You just have to adjust your perspective slightly.

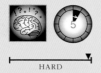

25 Sarah's Game

AIM This is a tricky exercise that will take all your powers of concentration.

TASK In the grid of letters below you will find the name SARAH written completely only once. It may be horizontal, vertical or diagonal but the word will not be bent. You must find it. To get a brilliant score you must also find a similarly spelled but totally unrelated word that is also hidden in the grid.

S	A	H	A	H	A	R	S	A	R
A	S	A	R	H	R	A	H	A	S
R	A	S	R	S	S	H	A	S	R
H	A	S	R	S	A	H	A	R	A
A	S	A	H	R	A	R	A	A	S
S	H	A	R	A	S	A	R	A	R
A	S	A	R	H	R	S	A	H	A
R	A	H	S	A	S	R	A	H	A
A	S	A	R	R	H	H	S	A	S
H	A	R	A	H	A	S	A	R	A

POOR
You couldn't find either word? Keep looking! When you've finished this exercise try ➤ Task 113

AVERAGE
If you got one of the words, that's not bad. Keep trying to find the other before going to ➤ Task 42

BRILLIANT
Got both words in less than the allotted time? Excellent! Now try ➤ Task 68

26 Crossed Uncrossed

MODERATE

AIM This is a game that is not only fun but provides a valuable exercise in communication by encouraging you to look beneath the obvious for the true message.

TASK This is a group game – the more players the merrier. Only one player, the leader, needs know the reasoning behind the game (which is given in the answer section so that you can choose who reads it).

You need two identical long thin objects, such as pencils, table knives, pieces of stick, etc. The players sit in a circle and one begins by passing the objects to the player on their left. The first player must say either, 'I pass these to you crossed', or 'I pass these to you uncrossed'. The leader will then either agree that the objects were crossed or uncrossed or contradict the first player. The second player then passes the objects to the left and again attempts to pass them crossed or uncrossed. Naturally the game has nothing at all to do with whether the objects are actually crossed in the normal sense of the word. Players will experiment with different ways of passing the objects trying to find out what 'crossed' and 'uncrossed' really mean. Their only guides will be the comments of the leader when other players accidentally get it right. Slowly, however, players will begin to work out what is going on and, as the game progresses an increasing number correct passes will be made. Eventually all but the most imperceptive players will have worked out the secret.

POOR
If you didn't work it out then you are too hooked on the obvious. Don't watch the objects, watch what else the players are doing.
Try ▶ Task 71

AVERAGE
If you got the idea after a while, well done. Next time you can be the leader and sit there smugly while others struggle.
Try ▶ Task 63

BRILLIANT
If you got this immediately (and without having played the game before) you are very perceptive and able to avoid distractions in order to get at the heart of the matter.
Try ▶ Task 95

HELP
No, there's no help here. Just watch what's happening very carefully.

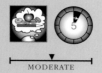

MODERATE

27 Lunch Bunch

AIM This is a simple task that will test your memory.

TASK The diagram shows a seating plan. It names 10 friends who met for lunch and describes what each ate. Study it for five minutes and then cover the diagram and answer the questions below:

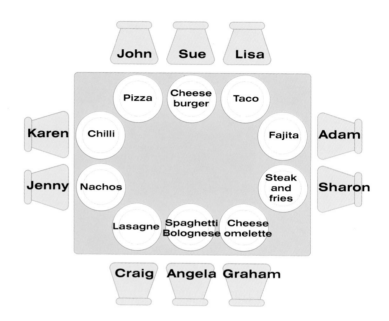

1. How many women were present?

2. What did Craig eat?

3. Who sat opposite Sue?

4. How many people ordered pasta?

5. Who sat to the right of Karen?

6. Who had the pizza?

7. Who sat on the left of the person who ordered steak?

8. Who sat between Craig and Karen?

9. What did the person eat who sat between the taco and the steak?

10. Who was diagonally opposite Lisa?

HELP
Try to memorize the table one side at a time. Keep closing your eyes and try to visualize the names and dishes.

POOR
If you got fewer than five your powers of observation are not great.
Try ≫ Task 45

AVERAGE
About seven or eight correct answers is a respectable result.
Try ≫ Task 31

BRILLIANT
If you got nine or 10 correct, well done!
Try ≫ Task 92

28 Word Wheel

AIM This is quite a tough test of verbal dexterity. It will take a lot of patience to get it right.

TASK What you have to do is fit the letters below into the grid provided. Put one letter in each segment and one in the circle in the centre. You must end up with nine five-letter words all ending with the same letter. If you've got it right the initial letters of the words will form the name of a plant with seasonal connections.

HARD

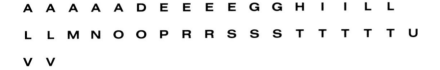

A A A A A D E E E G G H I I L L
L L M N O O P R R S S T T T T U
V V

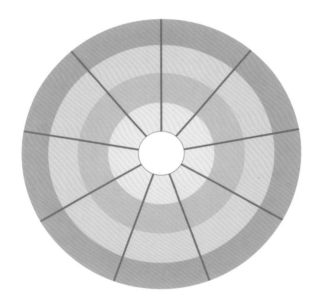

POOR
If you're not a word fan you might have run out of steam before solving this one. It's not so much difficult as very time-consuming. If you fall by the wayside try ❯❯ Task 15

AVERAGE
If you have the stamina you'll crack this one eventually. It's one of those puzzles that becomes easier as you go on.
Try ❯❯ Task 22

BRILLIANT
Word buffs will have solved this one well inside the time. If you do a crossword puzzle every day this puzzle should hold no fears for you.
Try ❯❯ Task 126

HELP
Think what that seasonal plant can be. Once you have that written around the outside the rest gets much easier.

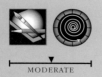

MODERATE

29 Candide Caper

AIM This riddle was thought up by the French philosopher, Voltaire. Like his literary creation, Candide, it appears simple but has hidden depths. As with all such puzzles the problem looks tricky but is really quite straightforward. Some readers will see the answer staring them in the face while others will struggle.

TASK What is both the longest and the shortest thing in the world, the fastest and the slowest, the most neglected and the most regretted, without which nothing can be done?

POOR	AVERAGE	BRILLIANT
Are you just too impatient for this type of problem or have you not solved it because your thinking is stuck in a rut? Try ➤ Task 51	If you got this within the time allowed your powers of reasoning are pretty good. Try ➤ Task 52	You may be one of the people who have a natural gift for this type of thinking. It's very useful not to have to plod step by step through a series of possibilities. Try ➤ Task 101

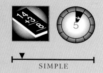

SIMPLE

30 Will he Win?

AIM This problem is not too hard but requires just a bit of lateral thinking.

TASK Augustus Rich had been a life-long patron of the Society for the Preservation of the Crested Newt. Over the years he had made many charitable contributions to the Society and always let it be known that, as he had no relatives, the charity would inherit all his estate when he died. Unfortunately, as Augustus got older, he became slightly eccentric and, before he died he changed his will to say that all his worldly goods should be sold and his money buried with him. When he died the Society contested the will on the grounds that Augustus had not been of sound mind when he made it. The judge was sympathetic and, being a clever man, came up with a solution that gave the charity all Augustus's money while obeying the terms of his will. What was the solution?

POOR	AVERAGE	BRILLIANT
Was actual money buried with Augustus or could it have been something else? Try ➤ Task 15	Got it at last? Well done. Try ➤ Task 57	Saw it in a flash? OK, try ➤ Task 99

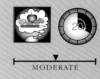

MODERATE

31 Association

AIM This technique is very useful for memorizing things like addresses and telephone numbers. What you do is find words or phrases that you can associate with the information you're trying to commit to memory. One of my friends is a very devout Catholic and was recently married. I remember her telephone number as, 'Oh heaven's gate, I do, I do, I do!' The number is 078121212.

TASK Here are some fictional names, addresses and telephone numbers to memorize. Make sure you use your powers of association to the full. Look for anything instantly memorable about each set of details. For the first one I have included some suggestions, but for the others you are on your own. You have 20 minutes in which to memorize the whole lot.

Graham Hopkirk, 27 Leason Avenue, Godmanchester 01325 283669
A grey ham hopping over a church. 3 x 9 = 27. Leason sounds like Reason. Think of God looking down on Manchester. The telephone number sounds like: Oh, one tree to five. Two ate three! Clickety click nine.

Sandra Farnsworth, 63, Glebe Road, Dorking 01592 967946

Harold Snoad, 47 Acacia Avenue, Wetherby, 01934 987024

David Kennilworth, 35 Barnstaple Terrace, Tewksbury 01759 672650

Alison Warren, 53 Culloden Gardens, Kelvinside, Glasgow 01538 686860

Caroline Fitzpatrick, 38 Darwin Drive, Godalming 01936 443957

POOR
If you find this difficult try having some fun with it. The more surreal your associations the better! Isn't it odd that Harold Snowed lives in Weatherby? Does David Kennilworth have a dog? Maybe Alison keeps rabbits in her Warren.
Try ⯈ Task 47

AVERAGE
If this one works for you but is hard going, keep working at your associations. You can add rhymes and bits of song as well, if it helps. The funnier and more memorable you make them the better they work.
Try ⯈ Task 73

BRILLIANT
If this one came naturally to you it will be an excellent tool for the future.
Try ⯈ Task 115

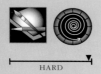

HARD

32 Chaos Controlled

AIM Many of our creativity tasks have involved coaxing flashes of inspiration to rise up out of the subconscious. This is sometimes all you need, but frequently the conscious mind plays a vital role in organizing this material into a useful form. That is what this task is all about.

TASK Start by setting yourself a task. It could be writing a story, solving a problem, planning some job around the house or anything else that requires creative input. Phase one involves jotting down all your ideas just as they come to you. Don't worry about creating a logical order at this stage. Just chuck everything down higgledy-piggledy. A computer is useful for this sort of thing but, if you don't have one, a sheet of paper will be fine.

Phase two involves trying to organize your thoughts in broad sections. This will give your project a structure or framework on which you can put the fine detail. Trying to martial your original thoughts into sections will inevitably lead to discarding some of your ideas as useless but it will also lead you on to new ones. You might find as you go on that you need to rename and re-order your sections so that your ideas make better sense.

The detailed work begins in phase three. Within each section organize your ideas logically so they flow in a way that makes perfect sense. This is especially important if your project is of the type that needs to be communicated to others.

This entire process is one of re-organizing and refining your ideas until you have produced the clearest and most complete statement possible of what you are trying to achieve.

HELP
Even when you have your project supposedly finished, always leave some room for the element of serendipity or happy accident. Your creative mind doesn't stop working just because you have consciously put everything in order. Be prepared at the last minute to dispense with some things and put new material in if you have a flash of inspiration. Usually these last minute changes are the things that turn your work into something special.

POOR
Not having much luck? Go back to the ideas stage and give that some more attention. Organizing can be tricky but the really hard bit is to have something worth organizing in the first place. When you've finished try ➤ Task 62

AVERAGE
When you've finished your planning, take a critical look at it. There are few really new ideas but does yours add anything to the way it has been done before? Is it more informative, more entertaining, easier to follow? Try ➤ Task 75

BRILLIANT
If you've produced a really good piece of work that satisfies you, then that's excellent. Try ➤ Task 8

33 Box Clever

AIM This is one of those puzzles where you have to pick up an image in your mind and manipulate it. Alternatively you can cheat and make the cube out of paper! Try it the hard way first. Many people (even those who are good at IQ-type questions) find this sort of mental manipulation tricky.

TASK Look at the diagram of an unfolded box. How many of the boxes below could be made from it?

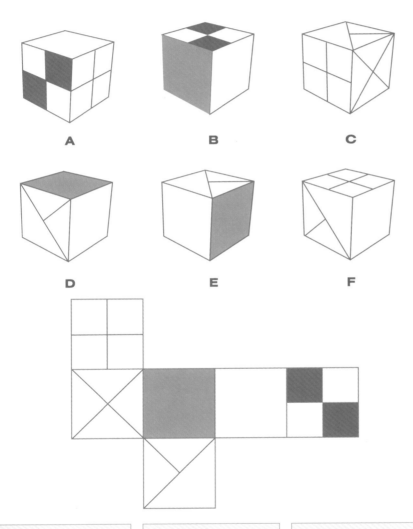

MODERATE

A   B   C

D   E   F

POOR
If you couldn't do this don't feel too badly. These visual puzzles take a certain special skill. Try ❱❱ Task 68

AVERAGE
If you struggled and won, try ❱❱ Task 40

BRILLIANT
If you're a natural at this sort of thing try ❱❱ Task 44

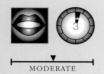

MODERATE

34 Between the Lines

AIM This is another game to improve your communication skills. It relies on players being able to 'read between the lines'.

TASK Two players pick a topic and begin to talk about it in as oblique a way as possible. The others have to guess what they're discussing. Take this exchange, for example:

'Did you ever do it?'

'Yes, I enjoyed it a lot at first but later I wondered if I was doing it too much and maybe it would affect my health.'

'Don't they say it's supposed to make you less stressed?'

'Yes, but I found I was gaining weight…'

Carry on until someone guesses what's going on. The skill for the talkers is to keep going without intentionally misleading the guessers but trying to be as obscure as possible. (In case you were wondering, the conversation above was about eating chocolate.)

POOR Think your way around the subject. Try ❱❱ Task 26	**AVERAGE** As you continue the speakers will get more subtle and so will the guessers. Try ❱❱ Task 107	**BRILLIANT** If you enjoyed this try ❱❱ Task 95

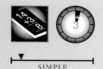

SIMPLE

35 What's in a Name?

AIM This is a simple test of your verbal reasoning ability.

TASK What do the following words have in common?

ARMY   TEAK   YACHT   HURT   SAIL

POOR Didn't get it? Try ❱❱ Task 50	**AVERAGE** Got it within the time allowed? Try something tougher. Try ❱❱ Task 53	**BRILLIANT** Got it immediately? Try a real toughie. Try ❱❱ Task 78

Doing the task Many word puzzles depend on anagrams. It's always worth checking to see whether the words supplied can be rearranged in some meaningful way.

36 Cross Quiz

AIM This is really a straightforward piece of logic if you don't let yourself be scared off by the wording.

TASK John is now just one and a third times as old as he was when he built his house and little Ben, who was 3⅓ years old when John built the house, is now two years more than half as old as John's wife, Kate, was when John built the house, so that when little Ben is as old as John was when he built the house, their three ages combined will add up to 100 years. How old is Ben?

HARD

POOR
If you couldn't do this you deserve a lot of sympathy. It's very tough.
Try ❱ Task 102

AVERAGE
Got it eventually? Excellent! That was a hard one and you did well even if you only cracked it in overtime.
Try ❱ Task 51

BRILLIANT
If this was the work of a moment for you, then you're a very clever person. Not to mention scary.
Try ❱ Task 56

Doing the task No tricks, just a lot of persistence.

37 Lucid Dreaming

AIM A lucid dream is one in which the dreamer is fully aware that what is being experienced is 'only a dream'. Once this happens the dreamer is liberated and able to enjoy all sorts of exciting experiences (unaided flying, for example) without any risk whatever. The practical value of lucid dreaming is sometimes questioned but, on the other hand, it's a heck of a lot of fun and very relaxing.

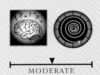

MODERATE

TASK First, start by keeping a diary of your dreams. This needn't be long or complicated, just a brief list of the edited highlights (this will also come in handy for the Creativity exercises elsewhere in this book). By keeping a record you will focus your attention on your dreams and keep them close to the surface of your mind. Next, agree with yourself on a sign that you will use to warn yourself when you realize you're dreaming. This could be anything at all, for example, tugging an earlobe or scratching your head. As soon as it occurs to you that you are dreaming, confirm it by using your sign.

HELP
The best way to become a lucid dreamer is to think of yourself as one and to go to sleep each night with that thought at the forefront of your mind.

POOR
This is only useful as a recreational technique.
Try ❱ Task 39

AVERAGE
Keep trying and you will get better.
Try ❱ Task 98

BRILLIANT
Try ❱ Task 57

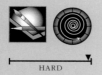

HARD

38 A Better Mousetrap

AIM It is said that if you build a better mousetrap the world will beat a path to your door. So do it.

TASK The point about the traditional mousetrap is that it is cheap, simple, quick and deadly. It's a hard act to follow and plenty of people have tried. The one below, for example, catches the mouse alive so that you can let it go in your garden and start the fun all over again. The task, therefore, is to use all of your ingenuity and mechanical skill to build a mousetrap. It can be one of those fantastical traps that leads the unfortunate rodent through a series of misadventures to its eventual doom, or it can be a straightforward trap that does its deadly work efficiently and, we hope, humanely.

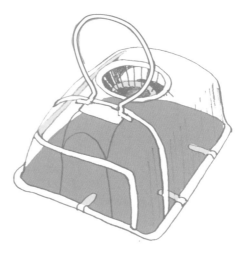

POOR
If you couldn't think of anything at all, don't give up yet. The very simplest ideas are sometimes the best. I once saw an empty milk bottle into which had been dropped a few crumbs of chocolate biscuit, used as a humane mousetrap that actually worked very well. If you really can't think of anything, go to
➤ Task **67**

AVERAGE
You came up with something that worked? If, hand on heart, you can swear that your device caught an actual mouse, you've passed the test even if your trap is not as good as the classic nipper.
Now go to
➤ Task **24**

BRILLIANT
If you actually did invent a better mousetrap you'll be off marketing your new product and looking for a patent.
Alternatively you could go to
➤ Task **52**

39 Mood Management

AIM Like most people, you probably take your mood for granted. Why? All you ever know is your mind. There is no outside to the mind so even your body is just a mind object. Mood is a function of that mind and it is changeable by an act of will on your part. Do you ever start the day by getting yourself in the right mood, or do you just accept that you'll feel grotty on Monday morning and pretty good on Friday? This exercise will help you adjust your mood.

TASK This exercise is most suitable for early morning. Start by getting comfortable. It is especially important that you should be warm, but not too hot. You can lie in bed, or sit on a comfortable chair if you prefer. Try a few repetitions of the Instant Relaxation exercise on page 97. When you feel relaxed, start to concentrate on the mood you want to create. A little background music will help. Think of the positive aspects of the day ahead. Think of all the things you will enjoy during the day. Have a look at your world through rose-tinted glasses and see all that is good about your life. If you have worries, try to picture them written down on sheets of paper. Mentally pick up each sheet, rip it up and throw it away. As you do this, assure yourself that you can deal with all your problems. Tell yourself that you are full of courage and confidence and that nothing that happens during the day will faze you. Think about friends, colleagues (the ones you like) and loved ones, in fact anyone whose help and support makes your life more enjoyable. Your day should now start with you in a happy, relaxed and confident mood.

SIMPLE

POOR
Try something new, if this exercise did not work for you.
Try ⇒ Task 135

AVERAGE
If you found this helpful you are ready to try a more challenging exercise.
Try ⇒ Task 77

BRILLIANT
If you are a natural born visualizer this could be a major addition to your mental repertoire. Try the advanced technique in ⇒ Task 74

HELP
We tend to take the mind for granted, a bit like the weather. It is important to get into the habit of believing that, just as you can redecorate your room just as you like, you also have power to adjust the set of your mind.

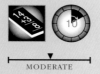

MODERATE

40 Fifteen Squared

AIM This is quite a tricky little numerical problem. Trial and error will, eventually, give a solution but those with a talent for mathematical thinking should be able to get there by a more intuitive route.

TASK Here are the numbers from one to nine positioned in a three-by-three square.

1	2	3
4	5	6
7	8	9

Your job is the rearrange them so that each row, column and diagonal adds up to 15.

POOR
Try working out all the combinations that add up to 15. When you have it try ➤ Task 97

AVERAGE
If you worked this out in the time allowed, that's good.
Try ➤ Task 88

BRILLIANT
If you got the answer in less than half the time allowed, excellent.
Try ➤ Task 44

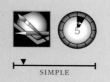

SIMPLE

41 Mumbles

AIM This is one of those games adults dread because they have to make fools of themselves for it to work. But it is the loosening up of inhibitions that allows creativity to come through.

TASK You need about six to ten people to do this. Sit in a circle and choose one person to start. That person must communicate with the person on his or her left. They can use gestures, noises, mumbles or facial expressions but NO words. Once the person being mumbled at thinks they understand the message they have to pass it on to whoever is on their left, and so on. After about five minutes, or when everyone gets tired of the game, each person has to write down what they think was being discussed and then take turns to read it out.

HELP
Play this game with some kids. That way you can pretend that you're making an idiot of yourself just to entertain them. But don't be surprised if they are more creative than you are.

POOR
Go on! Let yourself go! Pretend it's just for the kiddies.
Try ➤ Task 75

AVERAGE
If this worked for you then you should try expressing more complex ideas.
Try ➤ Task 106

BRILLIANT
If you really got into this then you should make it a regular part of your creative process.
Try ➤ Task 131

42 Kim's Game 2

AIM This is the same as Kim's Game 1 but with more objects.

TASK Look at the illustration for two minutes. Close the book and try to write down a list of what you saw.

MODERATE

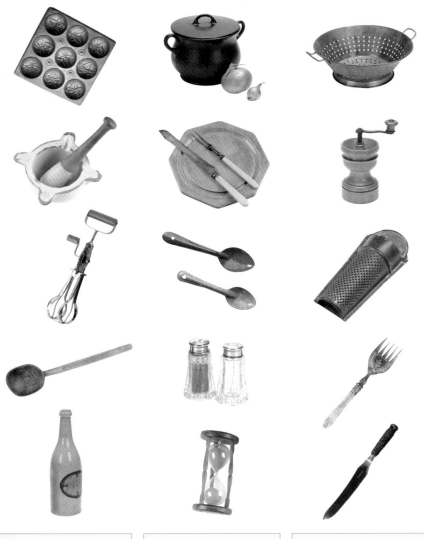

POOR
If you got fewer than seven objects this sort of memory is not your strong suit. Never mind. It is by no means the most important type of memorizing.
Try ➤ Task 135

AVERAGE
If you got 10–12 of the 15 objects that it a good effort.
Try ➤ Task 30

BRILLIANT
If you managed 13–15 of the objects, try the really difficult version in ➤ Task 87

HELP
Don't try to learn the objects as you would learn facts for a test. All you need here is very short-term memory. Just look at your mental image and check off each object as you see it. If your visual imagination is good, take each object in your mind's eye and throw it over your shoulder as you name it.

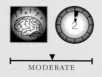

MODERATE

43 Following the Breath

AIM This is an extremely powerful form of meditation that has its origins in Zen, though here it is devoid of any religious connotations and can be practised by those of any persuasion.

TASK Start with the Basic Meditation exercise in task 3. After you have completed the breath-counting exercise five times, stop counting and simply follow your breathing. This might seem less demanding than keeping count of your breaths but the opposite is true. To keep focused on your breath without the help of counting is really difficult. The tendency is for your mind to wander but you must keep bringing it back to your breathing. Next, try to find your *hara*. This is a spot, a couple of centimetres below the navel that, if stimulated properly, will release a great flood of energy to power your meditation. Just try to feel that spot and, as you breathe in, direct the air to the *hara*. Create a gentle (repeat gentle) pressure in your lower abdomen. Once you have got this working properly all you need to do is follow your breathing without letting your attention waver. This may at first appear a very plain and boring exercise but do not be fooled, it is immensely powerful and, if cultivated properly, will bring great benefits in health, freedom from stress and mental development. Just as sitting in the cockpit of an aircraft can give you no idea of what it's like to fly one, so the early stages of meditation do not give you an inkling of all that you will be able to learn later.

HELP
Please note that once you have followed this path for a short distance, there is no turning back even if you give up meditating. There is nothing to be alarmed about in this, the meditation brings untold benefits but you need to be aware that it is a lifelong commitment and not a toy.

POOR
Not everyone is suited to this form of meditation. If you find it is not for you, then go back to the basic system with which you are now familiar.
Try ➤ Task 16

AVERAGE
If you felt that you got on quite well with this you must decide whether you want to continue with this practice. The benefits are great but so is the amount of time and energy you will have to invest.
Try ➤ Task 109

BRILLIANT
Some people just know that they are made for meditation. If you are one of those then nothing I or anyone else can say will make any difference to you.
Try ➤ Task 49

44 Small Change

AIM This is a test of visual reasoning. You might find it easier to try it with real coins.

HARD

TASK Below is a square with four coins on each side. Rearrange them to make another square with five coins on each side.

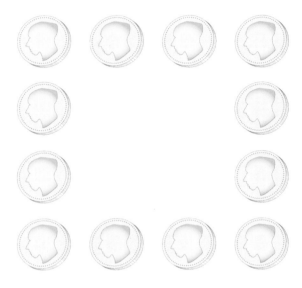

POOR
If you can't do it, think about this: you have to make a square but there are no instructions about what that square should look like except that it has five coins on each side. Have another think. When you've finished here try ❱❱ Task 22

AVERAGE
If you did that within 10 minutes your powers of reasoning are in good shape. Did it help to work on the problem with real coins or could you do it in your head?
Try ❱❱ Task 48

BRILLIANT
If you got that in less than half the time allowed and without fiddling around with real coins, you did really well.
Try ❱❱ Task 53

MODERATE

45 Pattern Poser 1

AIM This is a test of visual memory.

TASK Take five minutes to study the pattern below. Then, close the book and try to draw it from memory.

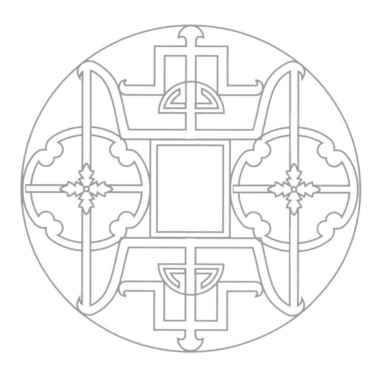

POOR
This is a test of memory, not artistic skill, so don't worry if your drawing is a bit lop-sided. The important thing is whether or not you can remember details of the pattern. If, after five minutes' study, it was still just a blur to you, then visual memory is just not your thing.
Try ≫ Task **62**

AVERAGE
If you managed something that was not too far from the original, give yourself a break and then have another try to see if you can get even closer.
Try ≫ Task **33**

BRILLIANT
Got it almost exactly? OK, now try another memory test.
Try ≫ Task **55**

HELP
The pattern is symmetrical so you really only have to learn half of it.

46 Code Breaker 1

AIM Most of the tasks concerned with communication are about improving your ability in this area, but a few are about defeating obstacles that hinder communication.

TASK Below you will find a message in code. Your task is to crack it. The code in question was invented by a secret society called the Rosicrucians and for centuries it remained secure. Even now, if you weren't given some help, you might find it too hard to crack. So look at the two diagrams below the code. They play a vital part in cracking it. Here's the message:

HARD

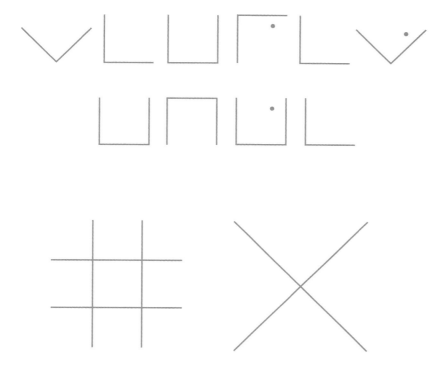

POOR
If you haven't cracked it yet think about the diagrams again. When you have finished try » Task 71

AVERAGE
If you got this after some head scratching, well done. There is another code in » Task 107

BRILLIANT
If you did this easily, go to the much harder exercise in » Task 72

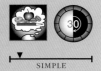

SIMPLE

47 Repetition Repetition Repetition

AIM Repetition is probably the simplest and oldest memory device, but that doesn't mean you should fail to take advantage of it.

TASK Simply repeating something over and over to yourself will help to create a memory, though probably not a long-lasting one. The school kid's trick of learning spellings or multiplication tables last thing at night and then sleeping with the book under their pillow is effective if all you want to do is pass a test the next day, but the memory will soon fade. Sometimes, however, you need to learn something just for a short time and not be burdened with it forever. In that case repetition is an ideal technique. If you want the memory to be stronger, then combine it with one of the other techniques (such as rhyming or association).

Here is a little bit of Shakespeare (from *Henry IV*, Part 2). Repeat it out loud and then try it with your eyes shut. Keep doing this until you can remember the whole piece. See how long the memory lasts without any other technique to help strengthen it:

> O sleep! O gentle sleep!
>
> Nature's soft nurse, how have I frighted thee,
>
> That thou no more wilt weight mine eyelids down
>
> And steep my senses in forgetfulness?
>
> Why rather, sleep, liest thou in smoky cribs,
>
> Upon uneasy pallets stretching thee,
>
> And hushed with buzzing night-flies to thy slumber,
>
> Than in the perfumed chambers of the great,
>
> Under the canopies of costly state,
>
> And lulled with sound of sweetest melody?

POOR	**AVERAGE**	**BRILLIANT**
If you find it hard to make this work you need to reinforce it with some other technique. Try » Task 13	If this worked after a number of repetitions and the memory lasted for a day or two you now have an excellent tool for creating a brief memory. Try » Task 31	If you were able to do this after only a few repetitions and were able to retain the memory for up to 48 hours, then you have found a useful tool for improving your memory. Try » Task 92

48 Colour Conundrum

AIM If you know some physics this one will be easy – as long as you can remember the rules! If, on the other hand, you have to think it out for yourself, you may find it quite tricky.

TASK Three discs of coloured light are projected on a screen. Which colour would you expect to see where the discs merge in the centre?

MODERATE

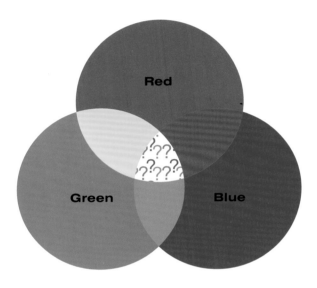

POOR
If you couldn't puzzle it out or came to the wrong conclusion, go back to the Help panel.
Try ▶ Task 9

AVERAGE
If you managed to reason this one out for yourself (rather than remembering stuff from your schooldays or looking it up), well done. Now reward yourself with
▶ Task 2

BRILLIANT
If the answer was apparent right away, that's great.
Try ▶ Task 120

HELP
Think about a prism. Does that help?

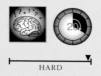

HARD

49 Chakra Meditation

AIM This is an Indian meditation system that relies on seven chakras or energy centres that correspond roughly to the main endocrine glands. The aim is to stimulate each centre and release its energy.

TASK Before attempting this you need to work on Basic Meditation on page 13. To start chakra meditation you begin as usual with counting your breaths. After five repetitions you can stop counting and begin to concentrate on the lowest of the chakras (see diagram). A warm glow should spread through the affected region. Once you get proficient at this, move to the next chakra and so on until you reach the final one on the crown of the head. Each chakra is associated with a particular aspect of the personality. These are:

1. **Root**: Base of spine – Survival, grounding

2. **Sacral:** Abdomen, genitals, lower back – Sexuality, emotions, desire

3. **Solar plexus:** Solar plexus – Power, will

4. **Heart:** Central chest – Love, relationships

5. **Throat:** Throat – Communication

6. **Brow:** Brow – Intuition, imagination

7. **Crown:** Top of head – Awareness

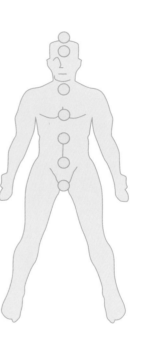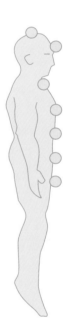

HELP
This is a technique that will take a lifetime to perfect, so don't expect rapid results. Try to practise every day and you will find that, little by little, your ability increases.

POOR
This exercise is not suitable for everyone so, if you find it hard, try one of the other techniques in ➤ Task 21

AVERAGE
Chakra meditation requires much effort and persistence. If you can do it but find it hard you need to decide whether it is worth persisting or switching to another technique. Try ➤ Task 43

BRILLIANT
If you find this technique beneficial you might also like to try Mandala Meditation in ➤ Task 18

50 Trump Trick

SIMPLE

AIM This is a non-verbal reasoning puzzle. It requires you to manipulate a simple shape. You can do this either in your mind or by cutting out a piece of paper and playing with it.

TASK Here is a spade from a pack of cards: What you must do is cut it into three pieces that will fit together to make a heart. You must use all the pieces. It's no good chopping the tail off and throwing it away!

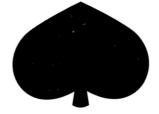

POOR
Couldn't do it? Try another simple visual exercise in ⇒ Task 91

AVERAGE
Did it within the time? Well done. Now try something a bit more challenging. Try ⇒ Task 48

BRILLIANT
Did it at a glance? Let's try something much tougher. Try ⇒ Task 28

Doing the task Visual tasks are tough because you need a special sort of imagination to do them. Just as some people are good at numbers, and some at words, some find visual puzzles easy. On the whole, however, most people find this sort of reasoning the toughest. If this applies to you, then work through all these puzzles and you should start to get the hang of them.

51 Same Difference

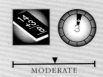

MODERATE

AIM This is a fiendish little task. Like so many puzzles it depends on a sudden flash of insight to get to the bottom of it.

TASK Look at these words:

BRING   BUY   CATCH   FIGHT   SEEK   TEACH   THINK

Apart from the fact that they are all common English verbs, what feature do they have in common?

POOR
If you couldn't crack this one try to think a bit more flexibly next time. Try ⇒ Task 88

AVERAGE
If you cracked this one eventually, then try ⇒ Task 53

BRILLIANT
No trouble with this one? Now try something harder. Try ⇒ Task 90

Doing the task If you are finding this one tough, it's better to think of sounds rather than meanings.

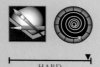

52 Mini Story

AIM This is an exercise in ultra-concise communication.

TASK The task is simply to write a whole story in no more than 50 words. Impossible? Certainly not. One way to do it would be to compose a longer story and then find ways to cut out all the flim-flam until you get to something that is both pithy and entertaining. Don't try this exercise just once and then give up. It will take most people quite a few tries before they produce their best effort. The more difficult, but ultimately more successful, way to do it is to use words like bricks in a wall when building your story. Build a bit at a time the way a bricklayer does, laying each brick perfectly in place so it can do exactly the right job.

POOR	AVERAGE	BRILLIANT
Some people will find this very difficult. But don't give up – it really is a valuable exercise. Try ➤ Task 6	Keep cutting! Cut until you reach bone and then file the bone down too. You'll soon realize how much a severe pruning will improve your writing. Try ➤ Task 16	Satisfied with your work? Try ➤ Task 75

53 What Next?

AIM Series puzzles can be fiercely difficult unless you are on the same wavelength as the person composing the puzzle. This one is a good example. The series takes an unusual slant on a series that you are very familiar with.

TASK All you have to do is complete this series:

O   U   E   H   R   A   ?

POOR	AVERAGE	BRILLIANT
If you didn't get this try ➤ Task 102	Got it eventually? Well done. Try ➤ Task 93	Didn't fool you for a moment? Hmm, the six letters in the series are a bit of a giveaway aren't they? Try ➤ Task 97

HELP
How many letters are there in the series? Does this tell you anything?

Doing the task If you're finding this hard, think of things that come in sets. For example, the names of the planets are often used, as are the months of the year. Also bear in mind that the letters needn't be the initials of words.

54 Deep Relaxation

SIMPLE

AIM This is a very simple but powerful technique for recharging your batteries. You may think that the end result (going to sleep) is easily achieved without any special help, but the sleep you gain by this method will be deeper and far more relaxing than any sleep you've ever had before. It will refresh you thoroughly, reduce your stress levels and make you ready for whatever tasks lie ahead.

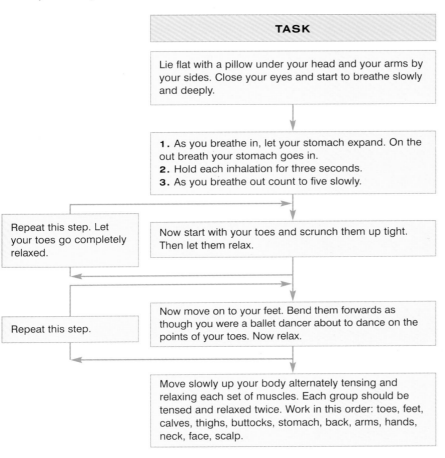

TASK

Lie flat with a pillow under your head and your arms by your sides. Close your eyes and start to breathe slowly and deeply.

1. As you breathe in, let your stomach expand. On the out breath your stomach goes in.
2. Hold each inhalation for three seconds.
3. As you breathe out count to five slowly.

Repeat this step. Let your toes go completely relaxed.

Now start with your toes and scrunch them up tight. Then let them relax.

Repeat this step.

Now move on to your feet. Bend them forwards as though you were a ballet dancer about to dance on the points of your toes. Now relax.

Move slowly up your body alternately tensing and relaxing each set of muscles. Each group should be tensed and relaxed twice. Work in this order: toes, feet, calves, thighs, buttocks, stomach, back, arms, hands, neck, face, scalp.

POOR
If you simply couldn't relax go to the breath counting technique in ➤ Task 3

AVERAGE
If you could do this for a while but then got fed up and fidgety, reduce your relaxation period. Try ➤ Task 112

BRILLIANT
Slept like a log? Woke up feeling wonderful? Excellent! Why not try one of the meditation techniques in ➤ Task 98

HELP
Choose a time when you are unlikely to be disturbed and when you naturally feel tired (early evening, for example). Make this your regular relaxation time so that you it becomes a habit. Always make sure you are warm (especially your feet). If necessary pull a blanket over yourself before you start.

Doing the task If you find it hard to let go, don't give up. People who find it difficult to relax are the ones who need to let go the most. Just go through the ritual regularly until you find it works. Very few people, except those racked with anxiety, can resist this method of relaxation.

HARD

55 Pattern Poser 2

AIM The following is an advanced test of visual memory. This time the pattern is less predictable and will require better memory skills than Pattern Poser 1.

TASK Look at the diagram below for five minutes. Then, close the book and try to reproduce it.

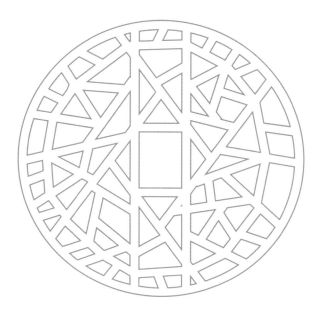

HELP
Try to get the main pathways first and then add the smaller bits as you go.

POOR
This is quite a difficult task so, if you couldn't do it, give up and go to
➠ Task 45

AVERAGE
Give yourself a bit longer and see if you can get a better likeness.
Try ➠ Task 27

BRILLIANT
Your visual memory is astonishing! You could have a great future as a spy.
Try ➠ Task 136

MODERATE

56 Pizza Poser

AIM Here's a little logical poser that might have you chewing a pencil instead of a pizza.

TASK Two mothers and two daughters went out for lunch. They bought a giant pizza and divided it into equal parts using five straight cuts. They then each had equal shares of the pizza. How did they do it?

POOR
Try ➠ Task 2

AVERAGE
Try ➠ Task 28

BRILLIANT
Try ➠ Task 36

57 Nose to the Grindstone

AIM This is an exercise in applied concentration. Previous tasks will have shown you how to boost your powers of concentration but now it's time to take your newfound skills and put them to the test in a real world situation.

HARD

TASK Choose a job that will keep you occupied for about 30 minutes. It needn't be a specific type of task. It could be anything from writing a letter to mending the car. The main requirement is that it should be something requiring your undivided attention. Now structure your time. Divide the task into parts (such as planning, gathering materials and so on) and decide approximately how long each part will take you. You can readjust your assessment as you go along if necessary. Add an inducement to keep yourself happy. Promise yourself a coffee break or a snack when you've finished. Now the hard part: once you've started DO NOT ALLOW YOURSELF TO BE DISTRACTED. Choose a time when you are unlikely to be interrupted by visitors or phone calls. Work steadily and resist the temptation to break off and daydream. If you encounter problems do not give up and do something else, but think your way through them until you have a solution.

POOR
Kept letting your concentration wander? Try a shorter period (even if it's only 10 minutes) and work your way up. Also try Candle Power in
➤ Task **109**

AVERAGE
Managed 15–20 minutes and then gave up? Practice will help. Also try
➤ Task **21**

BRILLIANT
Iron concentration? Well done. Try a really difficult exercise like
➤ Task **74**

DOING THE TASK If you had real problems, try again but start with a much shorter task. Judge from your first experience and decide just how long you think you can work for without getting distracted. Once you have found a length of time that suits you, keep practising and you will eventually be able to concentrate for longer period.

HELP
Try to work in an atmosphere that suits you. Some people need peace and quiet in order to concentrate, others prefer to have music or chatter going on in the background. Some can work quite happily on their own, while some need to be with other people. Look for situations in which you find it easy to concentrate and use them to handle other tasks.

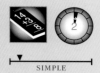

SIMPLE

58 Cubist Conundrum

AIM This is quite a simple exercise in visual reasoning. Even those who find the manipulation of shapes a bit tricky should be able to cope with this one.

TASK Here are several views of a cube. Can you draw the cube the way it would look if it were laid out flat?

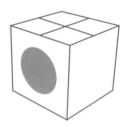
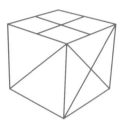

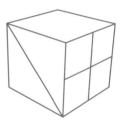
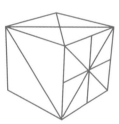

POOR	AVERAGE	BRILLIANT
If you couldn't get this right, then non-verbal reasoning is not your strong point. Try ➤ Task 99	Not too hard, was it? Try ➤ Task 33	If this gave you no trouble, try ➤ Task 48

59 Perpetual Motion

AIM This is a challenge for the mechanically gifted.

TASK The task here is to design a perpetual motion machine. Can't be done? Of course it can't, but that's no reason not to try. If you want a task that will stimulate those little grey cells and get you thinking creatively, then this is just what you need. There were many such machines created by gifted scientists that, at first glance, should have worked perfectly. The fun is coming up with such a device…and then working out how you got it wrong. Below is an ancient example invented by a certain Mr Fludd.

HARD

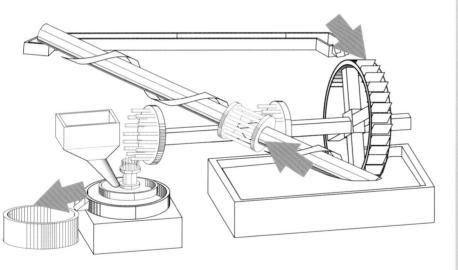

POOR
Couldn't come up with a ghost of an idea? Never mind, it was always the longest of long shots.
Try ❯❯ Task **9**

AVERAGE
You managed to construct something that looked convincing on paper? Excellent.
Try ❯❯ Task **106**

BRILLIANT
You cracked it? Hmm. Maybe you need to calm down a little.
Try ❯❯ Task **3**

HELP
There may seem no point in attempting the impossible but ingenuity knows no bounds. And, who knows, they said heavier-than-air flight was impossible until someone actually did it.

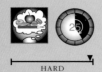

HARD

60 Memory Mall

AIM This is a really tough memory test that presents you with a challenge for your recently improved powers of recall.

TASK The diagram shows part of a shopping mall. The notes below give details of the shops and their owners. Take 25 minutes to study the plan and the notes (you may annotate the plan if that helps), then try to answer the questions.

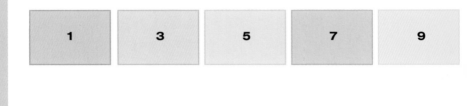

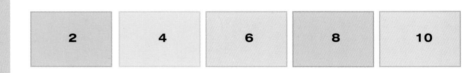

1. Mike's Bikes. Owner: Mike Marshall. Business established 2000.
2. Blossoms Florists. Owner: Jenny McCloud. Business established 1989.
3. A Piece of Cake. Owner: Juanita Garcia. Business established 1985.
4. Sparks Electrical Goods. Owner: Jay Williams. Business established 2002.
5. Dave's Plaice. Owner: Dave Green. Business established 1999.
6. Curls. Owner: Hannah Mandelbaum. Business established 1989.
7. Rick's Café. Owner: Jim Kenilworth. Business established 2001.
8. Carpet Heaven. Owner: Sam Quinn. Business established 1970.
9. Man About Town. Owner: Guy Needham. Business established 1976.
10. Gail's Fashions. Owner Gail Gonzalez. Business established 1997.

HELP
Try to imagine what the owners look like. List the shops in date order as well as by position. Annotate the diagram to provide a visual stimulus for your memory.

1. Which is the oldest business in the mall?

2. Which shop does Jenny McCloud own?

3. Where would you go to buy a carpet?

4. Which shop is next to Mike's Bikes?

5. Which shop is at No. 9?

6. Where would a woman get her hair done?

7. What smell might put you off your hairdo?

8. Which is the newest business?

9. Which business was established in 2000?

10. Which were the two businesses to be established in 1989?

POOR
This was a toughie so many people will get a low score. Give it another go and try to memorize more systematically.
Try ⏵ Task 115

AVERAGE
If you managed to get six or seven answers right you have done quite well. Try to improve your score with a bit more study before going to ⏵ Task 27

BRILLIANT
If you got nine or 10 right you've done really well and have excellent memory skills.
Try ⏵ Task 31

61 A Third Way

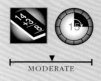

MODERATE

AIM The object of this exercise is to encourage numerical dexterity. It is not so much a trial of logic as of persistence. There is no quick way of finding the answer, but if you have an intuitive feel for numbers you should be able to get there within the time given.

TASK What you must do is take the digits from one to nine inclusive and arrange them in such a way as to make a fraction that equals one third.

POOR
If you couldn't do this at all, then numerical reasoning is perhaps not your strongest suit.
Try ⏵ Task 19

AVERAGE
If you struggled but eventually won (even outside the given time), well done.
Try ⏵ Task 69

BRILLIANT
If you found this a piece of cake then you clearly enjoy numbers and find working with them easy and fun.
Try ⏵ Task 78

Doing the task Bear in mind that the lower number must be exactly three times the upper. You should be able to estimate this well enough to rule out answers that are clearly ridiculous. If you keep answers that look about right' you should be able to refine your search very quickly.

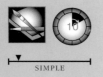

SIMPLE

62 Fantasy Faces

AIM Creativity depends largely on learning to accept the promptings of your unconscious mind. Inspiration has a way of rising up out of the deep unbidden but, if you are truly creative, you will develop the knack of seizing that inspiration and putting it to good use before it slips away. Here is one way of practising that.

TASK The picture below is of the fibres in some hand-made Japanese paper. If you stare at it long enough you should start to see images emerge. Faces are most common, but you may be able to find other things as well. See how many different ones you can identify and make a list of them. Be sure to turn the page around because you'll see different images from various angles.

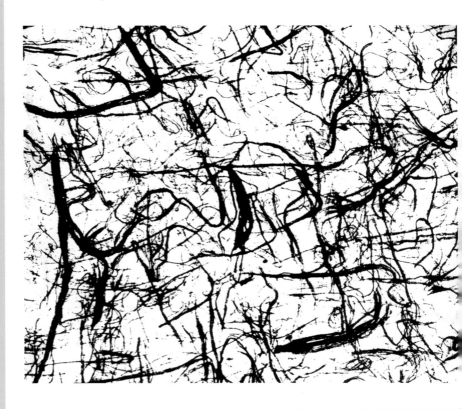

HELP
It's better to try this exercise before you get too far with the meditation tasks in the book. Advanced practitioners of meditation no longer see images in random patterns.

POOR
If you found only a few you are probably afraid to let yourself go. Take a deep breath (or even a small whisky!), and try again. Let your mind ramble freely.
Try ➤ Task 6

AVERAGE
If you found half a dozen images, that's not a bad result. But try again. Creativity is all about pushing your imagination to the limit and beyond. When you've finished, try ➤ Task 29

BRILLIANT
If you found that lots of images simply leapt off the page at you, then try ➤ Task 32

63 Charades

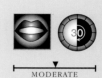

MODERATE

AIM If you thought that Charades was just a game to play at kids' parties (or adult parties when everybody is a bit drunk), think again. It is really an excellent communication game. It requires considerable skill to play it effectively. Most people have a passing acquaintance with the game but the method of play is re-stated here because it helps if you follow the system exactly.

TASK Start by playing the party game then, when your skill has developed, go on to act out more complex subjects. The basic rules are described below.

1. Tell your audience what the subject is. This may be one of the following:
   Book – make a book shape with hands
   Film – make an old-fashioned movie camera. One hand makes an 'L', as though holding the camera while the other winds an imaginary handle.
   Song – pretend to sing
   Name of person – pat yourself on head
   Play – draw theatre curtains in the air with your index fingers

2. Hold up fingers to show which word you intend to mime (one for first, two for second, etc.)

3. Hold up fingers for the number of syllables in the word. Hold up index finger and thumb slightly apart to indicate very short word. For long words you can mime syllables separately but hold up fingers to tell them which syllable you're on.

Useful signs:
   Tug earlobe for 'sounds like'
   Waggle outstretched hand for 'nearly right'
   Point at the person and tap your nose when they guess the correct word

POOR	AVERAGE	BRILLIANT
If you can't even mime The Grapes of Wrath give up and try ❱ Task 89	If you managed something as challenging as, say, 'Desperately Seeking Susan', keep going. A bit more practice and you'll get really good at this. Try ❱ Task 34	You managed to mime 'A La Recherche du Temps Perdu'? OK, so you're brilliant, but nobody likes a wise guy. Try ❱ Task 1

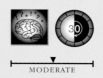

MODERATE

64 Self Hypnosis

AIM Hypnosis is a state of deep relaxation in which the subconscious willingly accepts suggestions made to it. Many people find the idea of allowing a stranger such intimate access to their psyche very disturbing but this method, in which you induce the hypnotic state yourself, avoids that problem. Because you trust your hypnotist completely you are much more likely to experience excellent results from the practice.

TASK Start with the procedure outlined in Deep Relaxation on page 51 Do not let yourself go to sleep! When you are completely relaxed you may begin the induction by counting backwards very slowly from ten to one. With each count say to yourself, 'Deeper, deeper, drifting down'. Picture yourself as a feather drifting slowly downwards. Now you need to create a sanctuary. This is a place in which you always feel comfortable and secure. It may be a real place, such as your childhood home, or somewhere imaginary such as sunny palm-fringed beach.

Once you feel confident in your sanctuary you are ready to pursue your goal. This could be anything from losing weight or giving up smoking to simply increasing your confidence. Always state your goal in positive terms. For example, never say 'I must eat less' but say, 'I shall eat when I'm hungry but not when I'm not'. If you wish you may use the Affirmations given on page 74 When you are ready to leave the hypnotic state wake yourself gently by counting from one to ten.

HELP
It helps if the induction is the same each time. Make a tape of your own voice and play it to yourself whenever you want to attain a hypnotic state. Be careful NEVER to use this technique when driving or doing anything else that requires your full attention, such as operating machinery.

POOR
If you found you couldn't reach a hypnotic state even after several tries, don't worry. Not everyone is a hypnotic subject. Try ➤ Task 112

AVERAGE
If you had some success with this technique, keep on practising. Also try Affirmations in ➤ Task 83

BRILLIANT
If this was really good for you, go to Affirmations in ➤ Task 66

65 Graffiti

AIM If you think that graffiti is just rude scribbling done by kids wearing baseball caps backwards on their heads, you're in for a shock.

TASK A major way to encourage creativity is to push the boundaries of what you dare to do. So this task is to go out and create a piece of street art (a much nicer term that lacks the negative connotations of graffiti). By all means use your own wall but if you use someone else's get permission first. Plenty of local authorities these days will allow you to brighten up derelict buildings by adding some art to the walls. Working on a large scale using spray cans instead of using a sheet of paper and some brushes will, trust me, be a liberating experience.

MODERATE

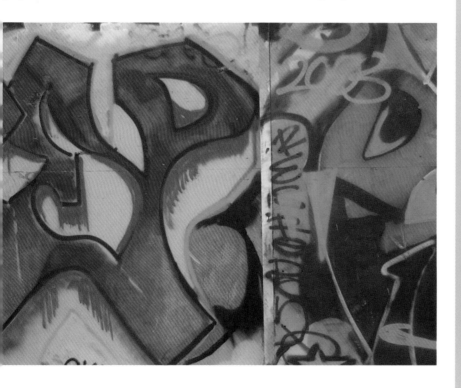

POOR
Didn't dare? Oh, shame on you! Tried but couldn't produce much? You can always white it out and start again. If you really insist on giving up, try
≫ Task 62

AVERAGE
If you enjoyed this keep at it. You can always use the same wall again and again. Working on such a large scale will give you confidence in all your creative endeavours. When you've had enough, try
≫ Task 106

BRILLIANT
A new street artist is born? Great! Why should teenagers have all the fun? When your muse is finally tired, try
≫ Task 38

HELP
If you've never done this before and are not sure how to start, look around town or alongside railway lines for some inspiration. You don't have to be 'good' at art. An inventive use of colour and texture will do a lot to cover up an ability to draw.

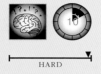

HARD

66 Well Well Well

AIM This is a controversial technique that aims to use visualization to combat diseases, including very serious ones such as cancer. The technique was, until recently, widely advocated not just by practitioners of complementary medicine but also by those in conventional medical circles. Recent research, however, has suggested that the technique is not as effective as was previously thought. There are still plenty of people who disagree and maintain that their own recovery was due to visualization. Give it a try and form your own opinion.

TASK Visualize your disease as a large block of some noxious substance (mouldy cheese, perhaps) that is being nibbled away by your body's immune system. The immune system can be visualized as a group of mice (unless you hate mice, in which case you should choose an animal more to your liking). As the block is slowly destroyed, visualize yourself getting stronger and healthier. Finish each session by seeing yourself happy and completely recovered. Repeat daily.

POOR	AVERAGE	BRILLIANT
This technique is not for everyone. Try ➤ Task 64	If you feel better when you use this technique, keep at it. Try ➤ Task 80	If you achieved real health benefits go to the next task. Try ➤ Task 102

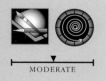

MODERATE

67 Twenty Questions

AIM This used to be a very popular game but, with the rise of mass communication and electronic entertainment, most people have either never played it or have forgotten how.

TASK One person thinks of an object, person, animal, book or whatever. The others (as many or as few as you like) are allowed to ask 20 questions and must then try to work out what their opponent is thinking of. This is a very useful game to play with kids (try it on a long journey). It is also good for adults who can, if they wish, play it at a more advanced level. The thing you think of can be as simple as 'cat' or as complicated as Heisenberg's Uncertainty Principle.

POOR	AVERAGE	BRILLIANT
Try to get rid of the impossible and then home in on the probable. Try ➤ Task 27	Keep this one by you for regular use. It will repay your efforts. Try ➤ Task 10	If you're a good guesser you'll appreciate the value of this game. Try ➤ Task 82

68 Bermuda Triangle

AIM Bermuda Triangle puzzles get their name because, however mysterious they look, there is always a logical explanation. This one calls for a simple mathematical formula that any five-year-old could apply. But, when you don't know exactly what is expected of you, it's surprising how hard a simple task can become.

TASK Look at the number around the first three triangles and work out which number is missing from the fourth.

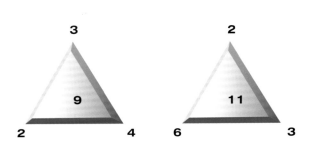

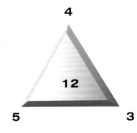
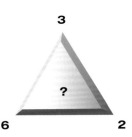

<table>
</table>

POOR	AVERAGE	BRILLIANT
Don't get it? Doesn't add up? (That was a hint!). Try ⯈ Task 2	Got it (but maybe took a bit longer than two minutes)? That's fine. Try ⯈ Task 15	No trouble? There's a tougher puzzle in ⯈ Task 44

HELP To get good at these puzzles you have to stay wide awake. This one is simple but later you will find that letters become numbers and vice versa. Stay alert!

Doing the task At this level it's all about looking for a simple relationship between the numbers.

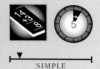

69 Second Thoughts

AIM This is so simple that you might just trip over it. Think carefully before you answer.

TASK The following numbers all have one thing in common. What is it?

2	1	8	8	1	2
2	5	2	8	2	5
2	9	9	8	6	6
2	9	0	0	6	2
5	1	6	9	1	5

POOR
If you had no idea about this one you were probably looking for a mathematical answer. The essence of problem solving is to keep an open mind and expect the unexpected.
Try ➤ Task 21

AVERAGE
Many people spend ages just on the verge of solving this one. The numbers look suspiciously symmetrical but what about the fives and twos? It is only if you think about the calculator figures that it finally makes sense. If you worked it out eventually, well done.
Try ➤ Task 33

BRILLIANT
If you have the right sort of twisted mind for this one, be careful, you could end up as a puzzle writer!
Try ➤ Task 80

HELP
Look for a twist. This is not strictly a mathematical game.

70 Brainstorming

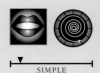

HARD

AIM This is a creativity task for at least two people (preferably more). It can be used for anything from solving problems to outlining a film, play or other artistic endeavour.

TASK It is important that a brainstorming session should not be allowed to become a simple committee meeting. We all know how much committees achieve. The idea is that a group of people toss around ideas completely off the top of their head and then try to use them to resolve a particular problem. The entire success of brainstorming depends on people feeling relaxed and uninhibited. If you're worried about looking like a fool in front of your boss or colleagues you will never have the confidence to brainstorm properly. A failed brainstorming session is miserable and destructive breeding nothing but frustration, anger and resentment. Be warned – make sure your colleagues are up to the task before you try this.

POOR	AVERAGE	BRILLIANT
If your group made no progress, give up right now. Try ≫ Task 66	If you had some success, keep trying. Try ≫ Task 65	If you have found a group that works well together you will all benefit. Try ≫ Task 32

71 Sketchy Thoughts

SIMPLE

AIM This is an excellent communication game and a lot of fun. You can buy an expensive version in a box but it can be played with pens and paper. The difficulty of the game can be adjusted to suit the players.

TASK The best way to play this game is to have one person make up a list of ten items that can be drawn. The rest of the players are divided into two teams and put in separate rooms. Each team then sends one member out to the list holder who tells them the first item to draw. They must communicate with their fellow team members ONLY by drawing. No talking is allowed. As soon as one item is guessed the person who guessed correctly goes to the list holder to get another item. The first team to work its way through the entire list is the winner.

POOR	AVERAGE	BRILLIANT
Don't be so feeble! It just takes a bit of imagination. Try ≫ Task 89	You enjoyed the game but your team lost? Never mind. Try ≫ Task 26	You were a whizz at this? Well done. Try ≫ Task 95

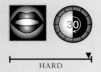

HARD

72 Code Breaker 3

AIM Here is a communications test based on your ability to decode a secret message. This offers you less help than the previous codes.

TASK The message below is in what is known as the Telephone Code. The diagram gives you a clue and, just to help you out, the answer is a song title. How quickly can you work it out?

3, 3, 8, 2, 6, 2, 1, 1, 2, 1, 1, 3, 1, 5, 1, 2

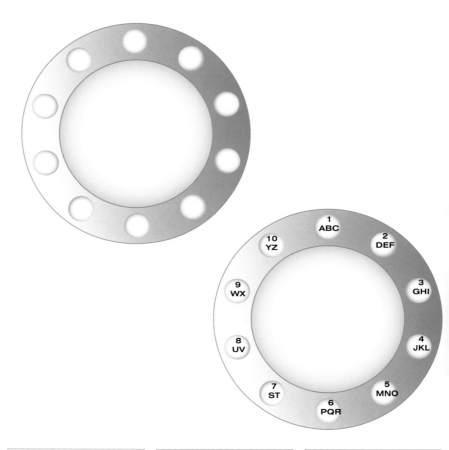

HELP
The telephone dial may not be the standard one you remember (assuming you're old enough), so part of the fun is playing with it until it works.

POOR
This is not just an exercise in logic but, like all communications problems, involves an element of intuition. How quickly can you get an idea of what is wanted? When you've finished, try ➤ Task **89**

AVERAGE
If you completed this within the time you've done well. Even if it took you longer, simply being able to crack it is an achievement. Like all problems, it gives way to a persistent problem solver. Try ➤ Task **107**

BRILLIANT
If this came easily to you, that is impressive. You have a natural talent for communication. Try ➤ Task **34**

73 I Remember You!

AIM One of the aspects of memory people most want to improve is their recall of faces and names. This task will help you practise that.

TASK Look at these children for five minutes and then turn the page. Do not return to this page today. Tomorrow (at the earliest) return to this page and, with the names covered up, try to identify each of the children just by looking at the photos. The ability to remember faces depends largely on intention. In other words, you have to want to remember the person. This is why we find it easy to remember people whom we find attractive. Another memory peg is distinctiveness. We remember a particular feature, especially if it is unusual. This is why it is often difficult to memorize the faces of young children because their features are not fully formed and, to some extent, look alike.

MODERATE

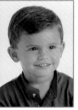 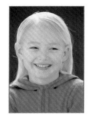 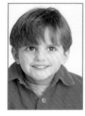 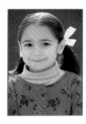

| Ben | Elizabeth | Sarah | Daniel | Nadia |

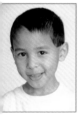 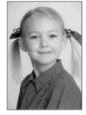 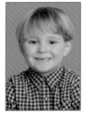 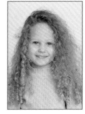 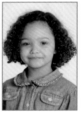

| Joel | Chloe | Max | Lauren | Charlotte |

POOR
If you could only remember a few names, have another try. This time, look carefully at each face and attempt to find some quality that attracts you to it.
Try ❯❯ Task 45

AVERAGE
If you managed to remember six or seven faces, that's not bad at all. With practice you could raise your score.
Try ❯❯ Task 10

BRILLIANT
If you got nearly all the faces right, try ❯❯ Task 27

HELP
We often remember people partly by context and find it hard to place them if we meet them in unusual circumstances. When you try to place someone it is useful to think not just of the face but of where you might have seen it before.

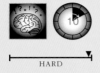

HARD

HELP
Don't forget that
your new situation
will have a down
side. In life there is
always a down
side. Before you
get too carried
away you might
like to work some
of these negative
aspects into your
visualization.

74 If I Were A Rich Man

AIM This technique is controversial but has many devotees who are convinced of its efficacy. It involves visualizing yourself in some situation that you deeply desire to experience for real. The theory is that, the more you visualize yourself achieving your aim, the easier it will be to bring about success in real life. My only comment is that, for the technique to stand any chance at all of working, your desire would need to be overwhelming.

TASK For the sake of argument, let's assume that you want to be rich (though the technique should work just as well with any other ambition you might have). Visualize every detail of your new life. What sort of house would you live in? What sort of car would you drive? What clothes would you wear? What holidays would you go on?

POOR
Not working?
Stick to a simpler
form of
visualization.
Try ❱❱ Task 11

AVERAGE
If you managed a
lengthy and
detailed
visualization, well
done!
Try ❱❱ Task 43

BRILLIANT
It worked? You're
rich? Don't forget
where you got the
secret!
Try ❱❱ Task 123

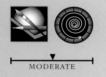

MODERATE

75 Doodlebug

AIM We tend to think of doodling as a way of passing the time when we're bored. Certainly we've never actually been encouraged to doodle, but could it be that we've been missing out on an important creative tool?

TASK This task could not be easier. Just take a piece of paper and any drawing materials you have available and doodle. Really let yourself go. Cover the whole paper and, when you've done that, take another sheet and do it all over again.

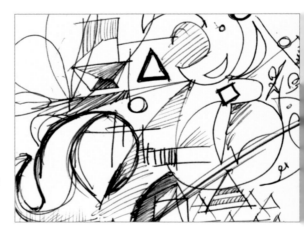

POOR
Try ❱❱ Task 10

AVERAGE
Try ❱❱ Task 28

BRILLIANT
Try ❱❱ Task 16

76 Tuning In 1

AIM This is a very strong memory technique that should only be used for information that you want to retain indefinitely. As a teenager I made the mistake of memorizing all my physics formulas to tunes from popular classics. I now can't listen to certain pieces of music (*Carmen* in particular is a nightmare) without remembering useless information about Watts and Ohms.

TASK Simply set the information you want to recall to a well-known catchy tune. For the sake of experiment, here's a list of the planets in our solar system in their order from the sun. If you're British sing the list to the tune of God Save the Queen (Americans can use My Country 'Tis of Thee which is, of course, the same tune). This is how it goes:

Mercury, Venus, Earth

Mars, Jupiter, Saturn

Venus, Neptune, Pluto

You'll find the last line a bit of a tight fit but that doesn't matter. In fact, paradoxically, because the tune doesn't quite work it will be all the more memorable. My father taught me the alphabet to the tune of Twinkle, Twinkle Little Star. X, Y and Z don't work at all, which is one reason that bit was the easiest to remember.

POOR
If you find this difficult you may not be a listener (see test in ➤ Task 47). See if Mnemonics helps in ➤ Task 92

AVERAGE
If this worked for you eventually, try a harder one in ➤ Task 45

BRILLIANT
If you found this dead easy, go for a complicated one.
Try ➤ Task 55

HELP
Always choose a simple tune you know very well. This technique is mental superglue, anything you learn this way is fixed for life, so only use it for really important tasks.

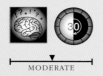

MODERATE

77 Insight Meditation

AIM It's a paradox that, although we spend all our time in the world of mind (for, after all, we don't exist anywhere else), we are also strangely unfamiliar with that world because we take it rather for granted. Just as you might imagine fish don't devote much time to thinking about water, nor birds about air, we are unfamiliar with the mind. Of course, psychologists are full of theories about mind but these are really of little interest to us in our everyday lives. What we need is a way of getting in touch with the mind as we experience it day and night throughout our lives. This task will help you to accomplish this but, first, you need to learn a simple technique.

TASK Begin just as you did in Basic Meditation on page 13. When you have counted your breaths for a few minutes, stop doing it and just remain quiet. Your mind will begin to wander and you should make no attempt to stop it. Just let it meander wherever it will and watch it as though you were a spectator. Whatever thoughts and emotions you encounter should simply be noted in a matter-of-fact kind of way. Don't push aside unpleasant thoughts or try to have 'nice' ones. After a while you should notice something interesting. Your thoughts are as slippery as eels. No matter how overpowering a particular thought might be, you are quite unable to hold it all the time. Your thoughts flicker constantly like a candle flame in a draughty room. Try to hold one thought for any length of time and you will find it will slip away.

Spend some 15–20 minutes a day at this exercise and you will start to learn some very valuable things about how your mind operates. You will find that certain thoughts and emotions predominate while others are quickly pushed aside. Some things you will think about most of the time (like it or not) and others you can hardly bear to think about at all.

POOR
If you find this difficult you might wonder why. Are you uncomfortable with your thoughts? What is about them that you dislike? Is there something troubling you that tries to bubble to the surface when you let your mind wander?
Try ➤ Task 37

AVERAGE
Ok, now try
➤ Task 79

BRILLIANT
Excellent!
Try ➤ Task 114

78 Maze Murder

AIM This is a task involving great concentration. The time allowed is short but, if you concentrate properly, it should be sufficient.

TASK There is only one way from the centre of the maze to the outside. Your task is to find it.

HARD

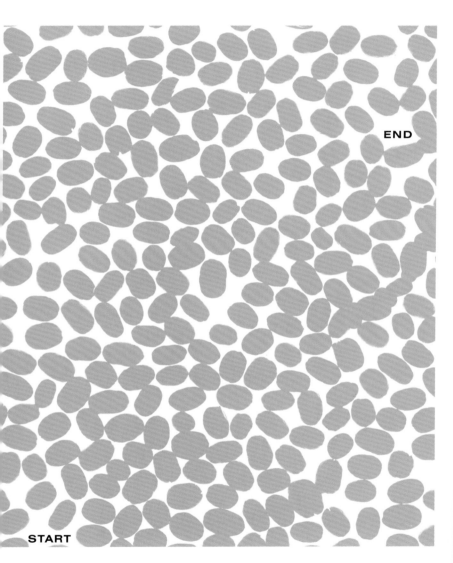

END

START

HELP
There is no magic solution to this puzzle, it's just a matter of following the routes as fast as possible to find the right one. If you concentrate fiercely enough you will get there in the allowed time.

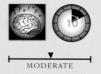

MODERATE

79 Just A Perfect Day

AIM Visualization is useful because, if you can see a desired outcome in your mind's eye, it is much easier to achieve such an outcome in reality. Some people find this so easy that they do it naturally without any instruction, but others find it very difficult. Anyone can achieve a degree of proficiency if they practise hard enough.

TASK Sit quietly and close your eyes. Start with a session of Instant Relaxation described on page 97. Make sure you don't go to sleep! Now, in your mind's eye, try to construct a perfect sunny day. Choose a location that you know very well indeed (your garden would be an obvious choice). Imagine it bathed in sunlight. Adjust your vision as you wish. Is it early morning light or that lovely orange evening glow? Mentally walk around the garden and see the flowers. Notice all the shapes and colours. Walk barefoot on the grass and feel it tickle your soles. Listen to the hum of insects. Watch the butterflies. Do you have a water feature? Listen to the water trickling softly. Feel the heat of the sun on your skin.

You can add any other details you want. Maybe you'd like to hear some of your favourite music playing softly from inside the house, or perhaps you'd prefer the laughter of children coming from a neighbouring garden. If you like, sit down in the dappled sunlight light under a tree and survey your perfect day at your leisure. Do not let any negative thoughts intrude. This is your perfect garden and worries or nuisances are not permitted to enter. You can even imagine a KEEP OUT notice if you want. Keep the exercise up as long as you like and, if you want, go to sleep when you've had enough.

HELP
Unless you know that you are good at this sort of exercise, you should prepare yourself by doing a few sessions of Candle Power on page 95. Try to commit scenes to memory. Fix details in your mind so that you can use them later on in your visualizations.

POOR
If you found you could hardly do this at all you need to work first on your concentration skills. If you lack visual imagination, cheat a bit and look at some photographs to give you ideas. Once you've improved try
➤ Task 11

AVERAGE
How long did you manage to keep your visualization going? If you kept it up for a genuine ten minutes by the clock, then that's a decent result. Keep trying because, just like memory and concentration, this is a faculty that improves with practice.
Try ➤ Task 42

BRILLIANT
If you found that your garden was luxuriant, full of delightful detail and you could live in it for hours, then try
➤ Task 109

80 Travel Turmoil

MODERATE

AIM If you get hung up on the appearance of this puzzle, you'll never solve it. It depends on seeing something a little beyond the obvious.

TASK On my way to work the other day I saw the following series of numbers in rapid succession:

8 -1 2 3 4 5 6 -7 8 9 18

Where did I see the numbers and why did they annoy me?

POOR	AVERAGE	BRILLIANT
If you didn't get this one, try ➹ Task 61	If you got it, try ➹ Task 84	Got it straight away? Try ➹ Task 89

HELP Where might you see numbers like this? What is that minus sign all about?

Doing the task I first set this puzzle for a radio show. You stand a much better chance of solving it if you don't look at the page too long! Think about the story instead.

81 To Boldly Go…

HARD

AIM Creativity is about going beyond the obvious until you get to some new place you've never visited before. This exercise will help you do that.

TASK Take any common household object, a paperclip for example, and try to come up with 50 (yes, 50) new uses for it. Why so many? Because after a couple of dozen or so you'll be struggling and then you'll really have to dig deep to come up with the rest. When you arrive at the stage when you feel you have nothing left to give, take a rest from racking your brains and do something different.

POOR	AVERAGE	BRILLIANT
If you 'just can't do it' then, sorry, but you haven't tried hard enough. Have a rest and then give it another go. Try ➹ Task 82	If you think you did very well but didn't quite make the 50, keep going. Really good ideas may come when you think there's nothing left. Try ➹ Task 106	No difficulty reaching 50 ideas? Excellent! Try ➹ Task 52

HELP Don't try to complete this exercise all at once. The trick is to push yourself to your limit, and then do something else while you wait for your subconscious to mull the task over. You can work at this over days or even weeks if you want to. If you persist you'll be amazed how many new ideas you can find.

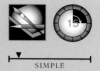

SIMPLE

HELP
This task provides two things of real value. First, the exercise will loosen you up mentally. By thinking freely you will break the bonds that restrain you from creative thought. Second, when you re-examine your recorded thoughts you will often find that the words suggest a train of thought that you can use in another context.

82 Free Thinker

AIM This exercise will loosen the grip of your conscious mind and allow those nuggets of creative gold from the unconscious to shine through.

TASK This is a version of the free association technique used by psychiatrists to help patients discover their unconscious motives. Here we are not concerned with disturbing thoughts but with creative ideas. First, make yourself comfortable. If you own a tape recorder, switch it on. Now pick a word at random and see what other word it suggests to you, then let the new word suggest another word and so on. For example, you might start with 'lamp'. From this you could go to 'light', 'dark', 'night', 'stars', 'travel', 'journey', 'adventure', 'distance' and so on. This technique works best if you don't think too hard about your choices. Run rapidly through a string of related words. The tape recorder will allow you to look back at your stream of consciousness.

POOR
Some people find it difficult to relax enough to do this. Try ≫ Task 11

AVERAGE
If you find this fairly easy make sure you keep practising regularly. Try ≫ Task 16

BRILLIANT
If you're a natural at this then your creative potential is great. Try ≫ Task 72

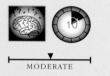

MODERATE

83 Affirmations

AIM Affirmations are little chunks of positive thinking that are dropped into the subconscious while you are in a state of deep hypnotic relaxation.

TASK Go through the hypnotic induction as outlined in Self-hypnosis in task 64. You can use some of the following affirmations or make up your own. Repeat each phrase several times and really work at meaning what you're saying. If you are using a tape to induce hypnosis, then add the affirmations to it. Remember to keep your affirmations positive. 'I will do better in future', for example, is far too negative.

I live my life with courage and conviction.

I live every day to the full.

There are no problems I cannot overcome.

My life has purpose and direction.

POOR
Not working? This is about belief. Try ≫ Task 112

AVERAGE
The affirmations get stronger with time. Try ≫ Task 64

BRILLIANT
If you find this helpful, keep at it. Try ≫ Task 109

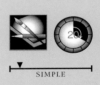

84 Fall Guy

MODERATE

AIM This problem will help with lateral thinking. Such puzzles ask you to step outside your normal mode of thinking and attack the problem from a different direction. It's a useful skill in all areas of life and, once mastered, can be applied to real world problems with excellent results.

TASK A man fell off a skyscraper and fell 80 floors without suffering as much as a scratch. He had no parachute, hang glider or any other device to help him. From the moment he started to fall, to the moment he landed, his fall was not interrupted in any way.

POOR
Didn't get it?
Try ❯❯ Task 19

AVERAGE
Got it after some thought? Now try a different one.
Try ❯❯ Task 94

BRILLIANT
If you found this too obvious try
❯❯ Task 44

Doing the task Take another look. Read the wording very carefully. These stories usually depend on some ambiguity or on a detail that you are expected to overlook.

85 Floppy Watches

SIMPLE

AIM This exercise is named in honour of Salvador Dalí, who is said to have invented it. As with most creativity exercises it provides a way of bypassing the conscious mind and getting at the unconscious, the source of most creativity.

TASK Just on the edge of sleep the mind finds itself in an area where the subconscious is very close and can be briefly glimpsed. The trouble is that you then fall asleep and probably forget everything you saw in this zone of twilight. The Spanish surrealist Salvador Dalí used to overcome this by using a technique in which he would let himself doze in an armchair. In one hand he would hold a metal spoon and on the floor he placed a metal dish. Just as he was about to fall asleep he'd drop the spoon and the resulting crash would wake him up. He then remembered vividly the strange visions he had just experienced. If you wonder whether it worked you only have to take a quick glance at his paintings. Now you try it.

POOR
Maybe you're not a natural catnapper.
Try ❯❯ Task 121

AVERAGE
If you got some results from this, keep working to improve your success rate.
Try ❯❯ Task 65

BRILLIANT
If this worked well for you remember to try it regularly.
Try ❯❯ Task 70

HELP
Don't forget to write your ideas down as soon as possible. Inspiration achieved by this method will evaporate like morning mist if not recorded instantly.

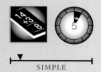

SIMPLE

86 Frustrating Figures

AIM This is an exercise in non-verbal reasoning. You can cheat by drawing it out on bits of paper, but you wouldn't do that. Would you?

TASK This square has been cut into bits:

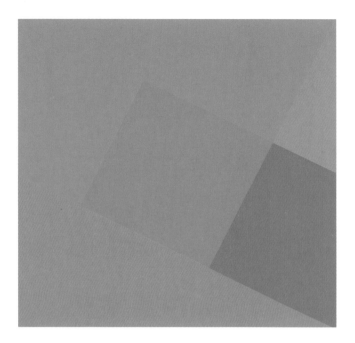

What other three other common geometrical figures can be made out of the same bits. Draw your answer but don't trace the original.

POOR
You didn't get any? You have the visual imagination of a log. OK. Cut out the little bits of paper and shuffle them around until you solve the puzzle. Try ⏩ Task 50

AVERAGE
You got them after much doodling? That's fine. Try ⏩ Task 33

BRILLIANT
You worked it out in your head immediately? Excellent. Try ⏩ Task 90

87 Kim's Game 3

AIM This is a really tough version that will test all but the best players.

TASK As before, give yourself two minutes to look at the illustration and then write down everything you remember.

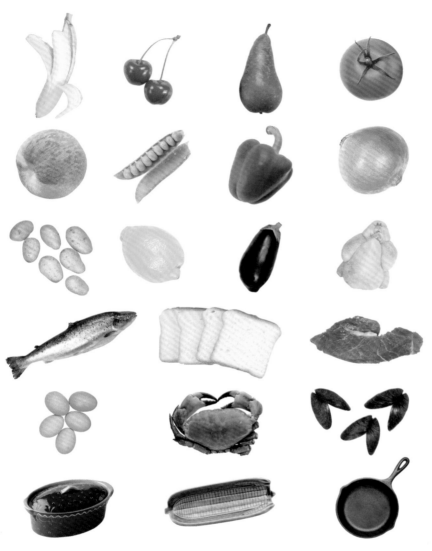

POOR
If you remembered fewer than 10 you need to keep practising. Try again and see if you can build up your score.
Try ➤ Task **14**

AVERAGE
If you remembered about 15, that's not bad at all. You can either try memorizing the others or try
➤ Task **115**

BRILLIANT
If you got 19–21 you are a phenomenon! Give yourself a rest and try ➤ Task **129**

HELP

In Rudyard Kipling's novel *Kim*, the eponymous hero practised this game until he was an expert. If this skill is important to you, then practice, practice, practice is the only way.

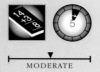

MODERATE

88 Match Mystery

AIM Matchstick problems are intriguing because they all look the same but are actually immensely varied. Some are mathematical, some are visual and some even require knowledge of Roman numerals to solve them. This one is quite special and requires a certain twist of logic to find the solution.

TASK Take six matches and use them to construct four equilateral triangles. It should quickly become obvious that this puzzle requires more than just shifting matches around on the table. Look for the unexpected element in the puzzle.

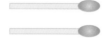
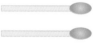

POOR	AVERAGE	BRILLIANT
No idea? Maybe your thought processes are a bit flat. Try ➤ Task 5	Got it eventually? If the answer came in a sudden flash of inspiration, that's your lateral thinking kicking in. Try ➤ Task 4	If the answer was obvious then you should be happy that your lateral thinking skills are so well developed. Try ➤ Task 44

SIMPLE

89 Forbidden

AIM There are many versions of this highly entertaining game and they all help to improve your communication skills.

TASK The basic game is very simple but the rules can be changed to make it as difficult as you like. First you write a number of nouns on slips of paper. This is where things get complicated. First, as well as the noun, you write on the paper a set of forbidden words. For example, if the noun is 'holly', you might have 'green', 'prickly', 'Christmas' or 'berries' as the forbidden words. In the simplest version of the game all the pieces of paper are put in a hat and then one player draws a slip, reads it, and tries to explain what the noun is without using any of the forbidden words. To make the game more challenging you can add more rules. For example, you can forbid players to use any word beginning with a specific letter. You can also use a time limit.

POOR	AVERAGE	BRILLIANT
Success depends entirely on your ingenuity. Try ➤ Task 63	Try the more difficult variations and then go to ➤ Task 6	If you've had enough fun here, Try ➤ Task 20

90 Lightfoot

AIM This is a real toughie. The instructions are easy enough, but the answer requires both logic and a good vocabulary.

HARD

TASK The letters below are all the ones you don't need to solve this puzzle. Work out which are the missing letters and then use them to make a 13-letter word. (The same letter may be used more than once.) The only clue is in the title.

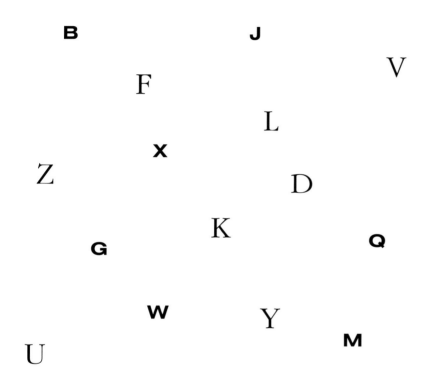

B   J   V

F

L

X

Z   D

K   Q

G

W   Y

M

U

POOR
If words aren't your thing you may not have managed to crack this one.
Try ▶ Task 7

AVERAGE
Struggled through? Well done. That was a real toughie.
Try ▶ Task 33

BRILLIANT
The work of a moment? Hats off to you!
Try ▶ Task 28

HELP
The best way of solving an anagram is to write the letters in a circle. This enables you to look at them in a number of different ways. If it doesn't work, try a new circle with the letters in different positions.

Doing the task Finding the letters is quite easy. The hard bit is turning them into a word (bearing in mind that some of them may be repeated). As usual, the clue is in the title.

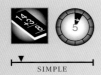

SIMPLE

91 Star Strategy

AIM Here's a test of your verbal reasoning. It doesn't require a huge vocabulary – the words involved are simple ones – but you'll need some ingenuity to fit the letters together.

TASK Take the letters:

L T R C V I B K A S B N E

and fit them into the spaces in the diagram below in such a way that you get five different five-letter words. One will read downwards, one left to right across the top (including the central circle), another in the same direction across the bottom (including the circle) and the others will read diagonally left to right. For extra merit, can you find a Russian hiding in the verbiage?

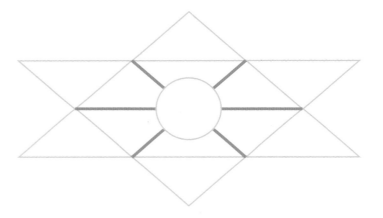

POOR
If you found this hard it's unlikely to be a vocabulary problem because all of the words are simple ones. Look for the common factor that links the words.
Try ➤ Task 9

AVERAGE
If you did this in the time allowed you can congratulate yourself and try
➤ Task 22

BRILLIANT
If you did this in a couple of minutes and found the Russian name, you're clearly a good verbal thinker. If you managed to make words other than those in our answer give yourself a gold star.
Try ➤ Task 44

HELP
All the words have something in common and when you've found it the puzzle becomes much easier.

92 Mnemonics

AIM If you are British you probably learned the colours of the rainbow by the initials of Richard Of York Gives Battle In Vain. If you're North American perhaps you learned the names of the Great Lakes as HOMES (Huron, Ontario, Michigan, Erie, Superior). You may also have learned to spell 'necessary' as Never Eat Cake Eat Salmon Sandwiches And Remain Young. These are all examples of mnemonics, simple tricks used to stimulate memory.

TASK Here is a bit of technical information that you will probably never need, but it will serve as a good test of your powers of recall. Listed below you will find the 12 cranial nerves and your task is to construct a mnemonic that helps you to remember them in the order given. First, divide them into groups of three. (Note that in each group I have put the shortest name first and the longest last, as this will help you.) Now make up your own mnemonic to memorize the 12 names.

OPTIC
OLFACTIVE
COMMON OCULAR MOTOR

PATHETIC
TRIGEMINAL
EXTERNAL OCULAR MOTOR

FACIAL
AUDITORY
GLOSSO-PHARYNGEAL

SPINAL
HYPOGLOSSOL
PNEUMOGASTRIC

HARD

POOR
Couldn't make it work? Try something a bit simpler. Pick another series of names that is a little less daunting.
Try ⇥ Task 115

AVERAGE
If you had a degree of success with this, then try to make up other mnemonics for yourself. Sentences can be fun. I learned the names of the planets as: My Very Educated Mother Just Served Us Nine Pizzas.
Try ⇥ Task 125

BRILLIANT
If you enjoyed this, then make up some more of your own, or learn some ready-made ones (of which there must be thousands in circulation).
Try ⇥ Task 129

HELP
For a really useful list of mnemonics covering a vast range of subjects visit Amanda's Mnemonics Page on the internet.

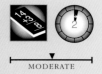

MODERATE

93 Ways To Learn

AIM There are three basic ways of learning: looking, listening and doing. Some of us (the lucky few) are excellent at all three, but others favour one and are less good at the others. It is important to know which style of learning suits you best. The following questionnaire will help you to establish this.

TASK Questionnaire

Answer all the questions. The answers that come 'off the top of your head' are most likely to be accurate which is the reason for the two minute time limit. Refer to the scoring key below.

1. You are learning to wire up an electric plug. Would you:
   a) Ask a friend to tell you how to do it
   b) Watch an electrician at work
   c) Take the plug apart and try to wire it up while referring to instructions

2. You are starting a new job. The office building is huge. Would you:
   a) Stop someone and ask for directions
   b) Study a plan of the building
   c) Walk the corridors until you manage to learn where everything is

3. You must memorize a long list of facts. Would you rather:
   a) Read them out to yourself over and over again
   b) Write questions about them on flash cards and keep testing yourself
   c) Write out the list several times to help memorize it

4. Which task would you find easiest:
   a) Learning your lines in a play
   b) Drawing a sketch map of the area in which you live
   c) Cooking a special dinner for friends

5. You have a new washing machine delivered and the deliveryman tells you how it works as he installs it. You probably watch and listen to him as well as reading the instruction book he gives you. Rank the importance of these activities to your learning by calling the most important A, the second B and the least important C.
   a)
   b)
   c)

6. If you want to remember a place you once visited would you rather:
   a) Read a book about the place
   b) Watch at a TV documentary about the area
   c) Eat some of the local food

7. If someone nearby wanted to attract your attention, would it be better to:
   a) Call your name
   b) Wave to you
   c) Tap you on the shoulder

8. Which would appeal most to you:
   a) A visit to the theatre
   b) A visit to a sculpture exhibition
   c) Attending an arts master class in which you produce work of your own

9. Would you rather
   a) Listen to music
   b) Watch TV
   c) Make something

10. If you go to a foreign country do you:
   a) Get advice by listening to people who have been there
   b) Find some books and look at pictures and maps
   c) Jump on a plane and explore when you get there

11. You want to buy a car. Would you first:
   a) Ask the salesman to explain the technicalities to you
   b) Look at some brochures and to get an idea of the models available
   c) Ask for a test drive

12. When learning a language do you:
   a) Listen carefully to native speakers
   b) Write down new words and try to remember their shapes
   c) Try to speak it straight away, even though you make mistakes

13. When explaining something do you:
   a) Speak clearly so that your listeners can grasp what you are saying
   b) Tend to draw diagrams or pictures to help explain
   c) Use gestures and facial expressions to reinforce what you are saying

14. If you were badly injured, the greatest loss to you would be the ability to:
   a) See
   b) Hear
   c) Move

15. If confronted by a new object would you first:
   a) Listen to the sound it makes (which is rather pleasant)
   b) Examine its shape and colours
   c) Touch it

MOSTLY As	MOSTLY Bs	MOSTLY Cs
Listening	**Looking**	**Doing**
Try ➤ Task 95	Try ➤ Task 129	Try ➤ Task 126

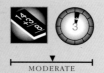

MODERATE

94 Clock Conundrum

AIM This is a particularly cunning puzzle that requires a combination of visual and mathematical skills.

TASK The problem is to take a traditional clock face and cut it into four parts so that the numerals on each part add up to 20. To give you the idea, our illustration shows an unsuccessful attempt.

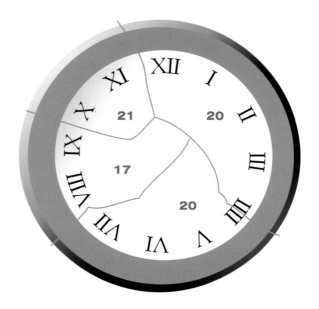

<table>
<tr><td>

POOR
If you didn't manage this one go to something more straightforward.
Try ❯ Task 9

</td><td>

AVERAGE
If you got this one eventually, then try ❯ Task 23

</td><td>

BRILLIANT
If this took you less than the allotted time, then try ❯ Task 90

</td></tr>
</table>

Doing the task There's no magic solution to this puzzle, it just takes a bit of perseverance.

95 Sixty Seconds

HARD

AIM For this communication game you need a quizmaster to control proceedings (which may become hectic). The rest of the players may compete as individuals or teams according to preference. The aim is to communicate as clearly and concisely as possible for one minute.

TASK The quizmaster picks one of the players and gives him or her a subject to talk on. The player must then talk for 60 seconds, measured by the quizmaster's stopwatch. A player who succeeds gets three points. Should the player hesitate ('um' and 'ah', for example, count as hesitations), repeat what has already been said or digress, then another player may challenge. If the quizmaster allows the challenge the new player may take over and complete the 60 seconds, winning one point. Other players may challenge should the new speaker commit a foul.

POOR	**AVERAGE**	**BRILLIANT**
If you're poor at this it is well worth trying to improve. Try ➤ Task 119	If you managed to get to the end of a minute with no mistakes, that's excellent. Play the game regularly until you can succeed every time. Try ➤ Task 1	If you are good at this, try extending the time limit to two or three minutes and use more difficult subjects. Try ➤ Task 17

HELP
You may have played this at school. Even so it is a valuable way to learn to communicate and is well worth practising. Keep a cool head and think before you speak.

96 Memory Lane

MODERATE

AIM This is a much more ambitious version of Around the House on page 115. It is useful for memorizing a substantial amount of information for a short time, for example, for studying for exams.

TASK Choose a route you know very well, such as the immediate area around where you live. Now divide your information into related chunks. For example, all your history dates would form one chunk and all your physics formulas would be another and all your geography facts would be a third. Nominate one road for each subject and, in your mind's eye, write each piece of information to be remembered on a board, just like a 'For Sale' sign. Erect each signboard outside a house that you know. Now lie back, and with your eyes closed, walk the whole route memorizing each sign and its piece of information.

POOR	**AVERAGE**	**BRILLIANT**
If this just doesn't work for you, then try ➤ Task 14	The more you practise the better you'll get. Try ➤ Task 10	If this works for you, then keep at it. Try ➤ Task 87

HELP
This technique requires constant repetition to make it work. It also requires regular maintenance in which you throw out information you no longer need and replace it with new stuff. If you keep this up constantly you will find your memory becomes invincible.

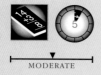

▼
MODERATE

97 Wonky Words

AIM This is quite a vicious little word problem that will put your verbal skills to the test. Anagrams are one thing, but an anagram with a bit missing? Hmm.

TASK Place one letter in the centre of the circle below. The jumbled letters can then be re-arranged to form words. To help you, the letter you put in the centre will always be the last letter of every word.

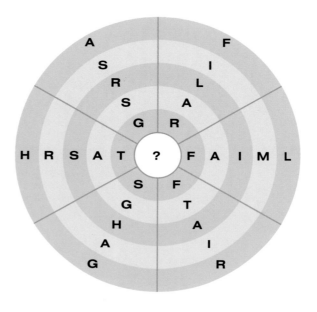

HELP
If you can't do this, consider why.

POOR	AVERAGE	BRILLIANT
If you can't get the answer, read the help box and sit in Zen-like contemplation until the penny drops. **Try ▶ Task 124**	If you got this within the time allowed you obviously have a head for verbal reasoning. **Try ▶ Task 90**	Saw the answer in a flash? 'Verbal' is your middle name. **Try ▶ Task 12**

98 Alphabet Soup

AIM This is a rather tricky concentration exercise. You need to keep your wits about you and, as the exercise progresses, the rules get more complicated.

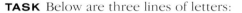

MODERATE

TASK Below are three lines of letters:

- In Line 1 you have to pick out letters that are next to each other in the alphabet (for example, you might find AB, DE, KJ)

- In Line 2 you have to pick out letters that have two other letters between them in the alphabet (for example, BE, TW, ZW)

- In Line 3 you have to pick out pairs of letters that have three other letters between them in the alphabet (for example, AE, LH, PT).

B D R S U W G K L J O Q S F N L

C E H K I J H R T V P M J H N Q

F J T X D K O R T O S W Z A E I

POOR
If you got less than 13 pairs you're not concentrating hard enough. Have another go and then try Sarah's Game in ➤ Task 25

AVERAGE
If you got 14–16 pairs, that's not too bad. Go straight to Sarah's Game in ➤ Task 25

BRILLIANT
If you got 17–19 pairs, go straight to Maze Murder in ➤ Task 78

HELP
Before you start it helps to write out the alphabet. Doing this in your head is just asking for trouble!

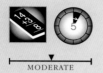

MODERATE

99 Penny Lane

AIM This is another test of your visual reasoning. It's not too difficult but the aim is to get you to use a bit of ingenuity in reaching a solution. **TASK** Rearrange the coins below to make six straight lines with four coins in each line.

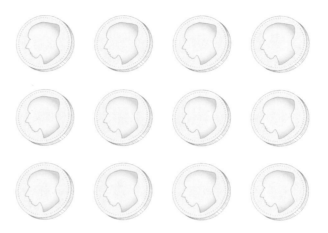

POOR
If you can't do this you need to understand that the same coin can appear in more than one of the lines. Try putting some coins on the table and moving them around. When you've finished here try ➤ Task 5

AVERAGE
If you got this within five minutes your visual reasoning is in good order. Try ➤ Task 104

BRILLIANT
If you solved this at a glance go on to try ➤ Task 104

100 Similar Circles

AIM This is a simple test of visual reasoning.

TASK Look at the five figures for no longer than five seconds and decide which is the odd one out.

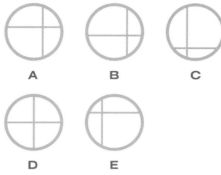

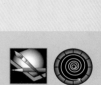

SIMPLE

POOR
A quick glance should make D stand out. If it wasn't obvious work on your visual reasoning.
Try ⟫ Task 58

AVERAGE
If you reasoned this out within the allowed time you're ready to try ⟫ Task 28

BRILLIANT
If this was a flash of the blindingly obvious to you, then your visual skills are fine.
Try ⟫ Task 78

101 In The Manner Of

AIM This is one way to try to break a creative block. It requires a bit of imagination but can bring interesting and useful results.

MODERATE

TASK Instead of considering a creative problem from your own perspective, why not take a mental holiday and try to work on it from an unfamiliar point of view? Here are two ideas: first, think of the problem as though you were somebody else. The choice of personality is limitless: Einstein (theoretical); Mandela (ethical); Lucretia Borgia (deceitful). Alternatively you could try placing your problem in another context and consider it as a game; soccer, American football, poker; chess. There is a wide choice of metaphors.

POOR
If this didn't work for you nothing is lost, it's only one of many techniques.
Try ⟫ Task 93

AVERAGE
If you found this quite useful it would be worth persisting. Explore other personalities and other metaphorical situations in which to place your problems.
Try ⟫ Task 8

BRILLIANT
You really got into this? Then work to develop the technique because the more you use it the better you'll become at it.
Try ⟫ Task 62

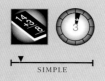

SIMPLE

102 Cola Conundrum

AIM This is a lateral-thinking problem that might cause you to pause for thought. Try to work it out in your mind's eye first but, if you get stuck, get out a glass and try it for yourself.

TASK You have a straight-sided glass of cola that is full to the brim and you would like to share it with a friend. You have no other drinking vessels and nothing with which to measure the depth or contents of the glass. How do you make sure that you both get a fair share?

POOR	AVERAGE	BRILLIANT
If you really can't reason this out, then start drinking and watch carefully what happens as the level of liquid falls. Try ❯ Task 19	If you reasoned it out in the time allowed, that's good. You get slightly less merit if you had to fill a glass and fiddle about with it until you got the answer. Try ❯ Task 94	If this one struck you as obvious then your powers of reasoning are in good shape. Try ❯ Task 90

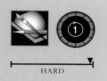

HARD

103 Egg Race

AIM This game is unashamedly stolen from an excellent television show that used to be hosted by Professor Heinz Wolff. It will test your ingenuity and allow you to compete with friends and colleagues. It is not only creative but also a lot of fun.

TASK To play the game you need a lot of household junk. From this you must construct a vehicle capable of carrying an egg without breaking it. How far the egg must be carried, and whether the competitors should be individuals or teams, are matters best left up to the reader. I would suggest that you start with a fairly short distance (for example, the width of your living room) and get more ambitious as your skill improves. Beware – this game is addictive!

HELP
Old springs or tightly wound elastic make good motors, pencil lead is an excellent lubricant, and bottle tops or jam jar lids are great for wheels. Using a hard-boiled egg is cheating!

POOR	AVERAGE	BRILLIANT
If you haven't got a clue, then maybe engineering is not the way you choose to express your creativity. Try ❯ Task 106	If you managed to construct a vehicle, however primitive, then you should keep working at this exercise. Try ❯ Task 29	Your egg is now approaching the next town at 60 mph? OK, you've passed, now try ❯ Task 84

104 Three By Three

AIM This is a fairly simple numerical puzzle. It requires no great stroke of genius, just a little logic. There are no tricks here. For example, the numbers do not need to be translated into letters for the puzzle to make sense.

TASK Look at the three grids. They all have something in common. Once you have worked out what it is you can easily calculate which number is missing from the third grid.

MODERATE

```
9  5  4          7  7  3
3  2  8          6  0  9
4  3  9          9  4  2
```

```
      9  2  6
      7  3  1
      8  5  ?
```

<table>
<tr><td>**POOR**
If you didn't get this one,
try ⇒ Task 111</td><td>**AVERAGE**
Worked it out?
Try ⇒ Task 44</td><td>**BRILLIANT**
Was it just too easy? OK, bend your brains and try ⇒ Task 36</td></tr>
</table>

Doing the task Once you see how the puzzle works you will understand that a five-year-old could solve it. Don't look for anything clever. The answer is just staring you in the face.

HARD

105 Name Game

AIM This is a tough puzzle because, once again, you don't know quite what is required. Are the letters a series? Are they numbers in disguise? Or is something else going on? That's what you need to discover. The task not only puts your ingenuity to the test but also the extent of your vocabulary.

TASK Study the following letters carefully. They are linked in a way that is not at all obvious. If you can discover the link you will then be able to supply the missing letters.

A   L   K   J   U   I   K   Q   ?

POOR	AVERAGE	BRILLIANT
This is a tough test so, if you didn't get it, don't worry too much. Try ➤ Task 108	If you got this one (even after the deadline) you did well. Try ➤ Task 118	Solved it in a trice? Try another tough word puzzle by going to ➤ Task 12

Doing the task Is this a series? If so, why are there two Ks? Maybe it's something quite different. Have a look at the title. That might help you a little bit.

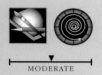

MODERATE

106 Bric-a-Brac

AIM Here's a simple non-threatening creativity exercise that anyone can do. It's really just to get you in the right mood.

TASK Gather together some household odds and ends (for example, nuts, bolts, egg cartons, empty yoghurt pots, those tubes from the middle of a toilet paper roll and, of course, empty plastic detergent bottles). Then use them to make a sculpture. How difficult is that? It doesn't have to look like anything and can be purely abstract. The only requirement is that you should find it aesthetically pleasing.

HELP
If you need assistance to do this, then you really need help. Try getting a three-year-old to give you a few tips.

POOR	AVERAGE	BRILLIANT
If you couldn't do this you're just not trying. Try again. If you can create something so appealing that you want to keep it (even if only for a while), that's good. Try ➤ Task 62	If your family liked your sculpture enough to want you to keep it, that's excellent. Try ➤ Task 29	If outsiders liked it enough to want to one of their own, you're brilliant. Try ➤ Task 38

107 Code Breaker 2

AIM Here is a simple communications exercise based on a secret code. This will test your ingenuity.

MODERATE

TASK Here is a message in code:

E2.A5.E2B4D3B3.E4.C4.D5.A1.C2.A5.D2.D2.E4.A3.B3.D2. B4.D3.C2.A1.D3.

How quickly can you decode it? Below is a hint to get you started

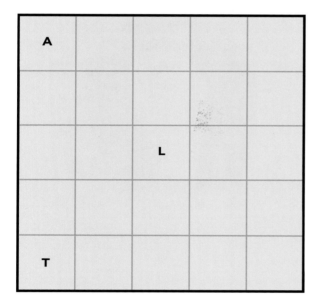

If you are really sharp you won't need to work out the whole message before you can guess the rest.

POOR
Still haven't got it? Traditionally the letters I and J were often regarded as the same letter. Does that help? When you have it try ➤ Task **89**

AVERAGE
If you've got the hang of this one try ➤ Task **26**

BRILLIANT
You can either try another code in ➤ Task **46** or try something completely different in ➤ Task **27**

HELP
This is mainly about context, both in terms of how the grid works and what the message contains.

108 Horseshoe Conundrum

AIM A mixture of logic and visual imagination will be needed to solve this tricky little puzzle. Like so many puzzles, it requires a flash of inspiration to work out just how it's done.

TASK Either visualize cutting or photocopy the image below and actually cut the horseshoe into seven pieces with just two straight snips of the scissors, so that each part contains a nail hole. You must not bend or fold the paper but you can move the pieces and put them together after your first snip.

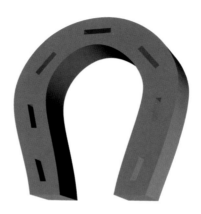

POOR	**AVERAGE**	**BRILLIANT**
If you didn't get it, don't despair. Try ➤ Task 113	If you worked it out eventually, try ➤ Task 40	If this was but the work of a moment for you, try ➤ Task 28

Doing the task If you're still puzzling, the answer depends entirely on the cunning movement of the pieces after the first cut.

109 Candle Power

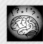

HARD

AIM This is a concentration exercise so powerful it is reputed to have miraculous powers. It is certainly the best way to learn this important skill. Once you have the ability to concentrate your capacity to learn and carry out tasks efficiently will be hugely improved.

TASK Light a candle and place it on an empty table in front of you. Stare at the candle for five seconds, then close your eyes and visualize every detail. Think about the exact colour and shape of the candle and flame, the wick and the hot dripping wax. Produce a really detailed mind picture and then, still with your eyes closed, see how long you can hold that image. This is very difficult at first so, as soon as you feel your picture has lost clarity, open your eyes, refresh your memory and try again. You should aim to practise like this for about ten minutes a day.

HELP
Don't be impatient for success. Aim to practise slowly and steadily. Many repetitions over a long period will be very effective but one heroic burst of enthusiasm for a couple of days will be quite useless.

POOR	AVERAGE	BRILLIANT
Try Nose to the grindstone ➽ Task 57, then come back to this one.	Go to Letter Pairs ➽ Task 122	If your concentration is really up to it try the maze in ➽ Task 19

Doing the task There's really no magic to this one, just lots of practice.

110 Toeing The Line

MODERATE

AIM This is a fun game that will keep people amused and improve their communications skills.

TASK Choose one person from a group of people and take him or her to one side. Tell them that, without anyone saying a word, the other players must be lined up in a certain order, for example, by the month or day of their birthdays, by house numbers, telephone numbers or whatever you can come up with. Even after the first round, when people have got the basic idea, it's surprising how difficult it can be to work out the order they are supposed to be put in and, of course, as the game continues the chosen reasons become more and more obscure. Astrological signs arranged according to their dates is a real killer and Chinese astrological signs are just for expert players.

POOR	AVERAGE	BRILLIANT
Your miming will improve with practice. But if you can't guess others' mimes you have real problems. Try ➽ Task 67	With practice team members start to build up a real empathy and can work out even very difficult mimes. Try ➽ Task 34	You did the Chinese astrology one? No need for you to hang around here, try ➽ Task 46

SIMPLE

111 Shapely Problem

AIM This is a very easy problem that has been made to sound much more difficult than it needs to be. If you read the question carefully the answer should be obvious.

TASK One of these figures is a set of all points in a plane at a fixed distance from a fixed point in the plane. Which is it?

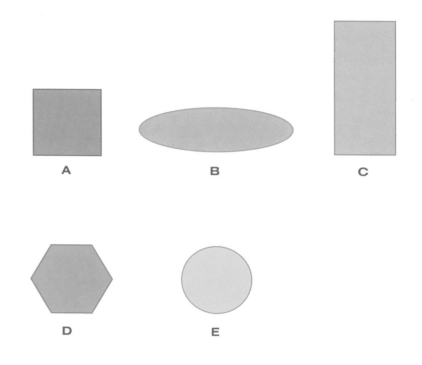

A

B

C

D

E

POOR	AVERAGE	BRILLIANT
You just let yourself be put off by a technical-sounding description. If you think calmly about what the words mean it becomes obvious what they are describing. Try ▶ Task 61	If you got it after thinking for a moment then you have nothing to worry about. Try ▶ Task 80	This should have been obvious so, if you got it immediately, don't get too big-headed. Try ▶ Task 12

112 Instant Relaxation

SIMPLE

AIM When you get tense and just don't have the time to do the whole Deep Relaxation routine (see page 51) this is a quick alternative that will help. You can do it anywhere, in the office, in the car (don't close your eyes!), even waiting in the last moments before an interview. It will also help you at times of sudden stress such as when you suddenly get some very bad news or discover that you've forgotten an important appointment and your boss is going to yell at you. This is not a substitute for deep relaxation but it's a good emergency measure that will help you to compose yourself in those moment of crisis.

TASK

Take a slow, deep breath.

↓

Imagine your body is the top of an elevator shaft and that the air is going in through your nose and then right down to the centre of the Earth. Feel the air going down, and down, and down as you breathe in all the way. (Yes, I know about the diaphragm but just do as I say and, with a little practice you'll get the hang of it. This is a very important ability to develop because it is used in the meditative techniques you will learn later.)

↓

Hold your breath for three seconds.

↓

As you let the breath out, count slowly to five.

↓

Keep this up for about 10 minutes or until your panic subsides.

POOR
This is the most basic of techniques so, if you couldn't do it or it didn't reduce your anxiety, you should take a look at your stress levels.
Try ➤ Task **64**

AVERAGE
If this helped then remember to keep using it and also try the more advanced Deep Relaxation technique in
➤ Task **54**

BRILLIANT
A lot of people believe that relaxing is something anyone can do, but it takes talent!
Try ➤ Task **86**

Doing the task Let your breathing settle into a nice, comfortable rhythm like the ebb and flow of the tide. Relaxation will come quickly but DON'T use this exercise to relax you so deeply that you fall asleep. When you hold your breath for three seconds, try not to let it become a strain because that will defeat the object. Hold the breath for a shorter time if that helps.

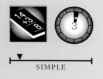

SIMPLE

113 Cubic Challenge

AIM Here's a chance to work on your powers of logic and visual reasoning. Unless you happen to have a lot of cubes and some paint handy you'll have to work this one out in your head.

TASK The diagram represents 64 cubes that have been stacked and then painted on all five exposed sides. Then some kid comes along and kicks the pile over. If you pick up a brick at random, what are the chances of getting one that is completely unpainted?

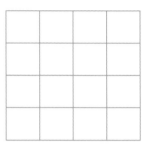

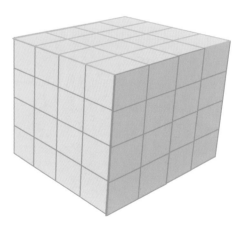

POOR
There is no real mystery to this puzzle. If you get it wrong you just haven't been careful enough visualizing which are the painted cubes and how many are left unpainted.
Try ⇒ Task **19**

AVERAGE
If you got the right answer eventually, that's good. Just a bit fiddly really, wasn't it?
Try ⇒ Task **26**

BRILLIANT
Didn't fool you for a second. Some people just have a knack for the visual. Lucky you!
Try ⇒ Task **44**

HELP
Count your bricks carefully!

114 Negotiation

HARD

AIM This is a more difficult form of visualization in that it involves a scene with other people. Their part in the scene will be to a greater or lesser extent unpredictable, depending on how well you know them. Even so, this technique can be of great value.

TASK Imagine yourself in a negotiating situation. This could be a multi-million dollar business deal (if that is the world in which you move), or something much less ambitious like discussing with a neighbour who is to pay for the storm damage to a fence between your gardens. Start by rehearsing your own side of the story. Marshal your arguments and visualize yourself stating your point of view calmly and confidently. Concentrate on not getting annoyed by the obduracy or aggression of your opponent. See yourself as calm, reasonable but utterly determined. If you know the person with whom you're negotiating well you should be able to handle their part of the conversation with some accuracy. Anticipate their counterclaims and think of reasons why they are not valid. Picture yourself politely but firmly rebuffing your opponent's views. Finally visualize a successful outcome to the negotiation in which you get a deal that pleases you.

POOR	AVERAGE	BRILLIANT
This requires a high level of skill so, if you're not quite there yet, don't worry. Go back to Just a Perfect Day, in ➤ Task **79** and use that exercise to build up your powers. Try ➤ Task **83**	If you could just about do this but are not satisfied with your performance, keep practising. You could also benefit from going back to the easier exercises and using them to increase your skill level. Try ➤ Task **6**	If this was easy for you, go on to Crossed Uncrossed in ➤ Task **26**

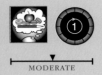

MODERATE

115 Tuning In 2

AIM If you enjoyed Tuning In 1, now you can try a real challenge. This exercise will teach you all the main bones of the body starting from the top of your head and finishing at your feet.

Human Skeleton

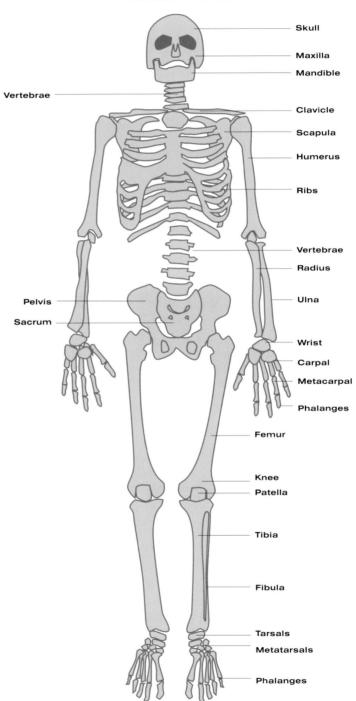

- Skull
- Maxilla
- Mandible
- Vertebrae
- Clavicle
- Scapula
- Humerus
- Ribs
- Vertebrae
- Radius
- Pelvis
- Ulna
- Sacrum
- Wrist
- Carpal
- Metacarpal
- Phalanges
- Femur
- Knee
- Patella
- Tibia
- Fibula
- Tarsals
- Metatarsals
- Phalanges

TASK I have set the information to the tune Dem bones, dem bones but, of course, you can use your own tune if you want. As you sing, follow the diagram and also touch the relevant part of your body to reinforce the message.

The cranium is connected to the frontal bone
The frontal bone is connected to the glabella
The glabella is connected to the nasal bone

Now hear the word of the Lord!

The nasal bone is connected to the cheekbone
The cheekbone is connected to the maxilla
The maxilla is connected to the mandible
The head sits on cervical vertebrae

And that is the end of the head!

The clavicle is known as the collar bone
The scapula's known as the shoulder blade
Top of the arm is the humerus

Now hear the word of the Lord!

Next we get to the elbow joint
The ulna sits beside the radius
And now we come to the hand!

The wrist is made up of carpal bones
They are connected to metacarpals
The fingers are made up of phalanges
And that is the end of the hand.

The sternum's known as the breastbone
It is connected to the rib bones
The spine's made of thoracic vertebrae
Now hear the word of the Lord!

The spine reaches the sacrum
The sacrum's connected to the ilium
The base of the spine is the coccyx
Now hear the word of the Lord!

In the front is the pubic bone
That is connected to the ischium
And now we get to the legs

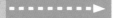

The femur is connected to the knee joint
The knee cap is know as the patella
The shinbone is called the tibia
This is supported by the fibula
And now we've arrived at the feet.

The anklebones are called malleoli
They are connected to the talus
The talus joins the tarsals
The tarsals are connected to metacarpals
The heel is called the calcaneus
And the phalanges finish the lot!

HELP
Using tunes to remember things is made even more effective if you tap out the rhythm as you sing, or even conduct an imaginary orchestra (though you might be a bit shy about doing it in public).

POOR	AVERAGE	BRILLIANT
Couldn't do it? Oh well, who needs all those names of bones stuck in their head anyway? Try the Mnemonics in ➤ Task 92	If this worked for you, even though it was a bit of a struggle, then it will be a valuable tool for the future. Try ➤ Task 87	If this really worked well for you it will be an excellent tool for the future but remember not to use it for trivial information. There are better techniques for that. Try ➤ Task 89

MODERATE

116 Delinquent Driver

AIM This sort of puzzle lures you into making false assumptions. All the information given is true but following the art of the politician, the story has been handled with 'economy'. Can you see the where the lie lies?

TASK Four young men were going out for the day by car. As they were going through a town the driver jumped a red light and crashed into an oncoming vehicle injuring its driver badly. All the occupants of the men's car escaped unhurt. Although it was clearly the driver's fault and there were plenty of witnesses about, none of the four men were prosecuted. Why not?

POOR	AVERAGE	BRILLIANT
If you didn't get this you must be every politician's dream. Always look deeply into what people actually say. Try ➤ Task 64	If you worked this one out eventually, try ➤ Task 88	If this was transparently obvious to you, well done! Heaven help the next ad man or double-glazing salesman who tries to pull the wool over your eyes. Try ➤ Task 94

HELP
Think hard about the driver.

117 Smelly Souvenirs

AIM Smell is probably the strongest memory trigger there is. The aim of this task is to use that fact to our advantage.

TASK The sense of smell cannot be used to memorize facts, figures, names, faces, etc. It would be wonderful if it could but, for one thing, humans are just not that good at detecting scents and, for another, memories evoked by smell are of a very different type. The sense of smell is excellent for evoking a sense of place. If you are of a certain age the smell of chalk dust will almost certainly drag you back to your school days and it is quite likely that a certain smell will remind you strongly of your childhood home. Such associations are mostly made unconsciously, but there is no reason why that should continue to be so. When you go to new places make yourself consciously aware of how they smell. Take deep breaths and savour the local scent (which, in the case of my fen village, involves large doses of pig manure). You'll find that these smells will act as memory pegs on which you can hang records of your life. It is amazing how a smell will bring back not just a place but the people and events associated with it.

POOR
If this doesn't do much for you, it may be that your sense of smell is not well developed. Some people are more sensitive to smells than others.
Try ⇒ Task 115

AVERAGE
If you've had some success with this technique, keep working at it. The more you sniff, the more subtle smells you'll detect and the better you'll be at tying in your memories to the various odours.
Try ⇒ Task 27

BRILLIANT
If you have a natural talent for scent recognition you must work at developing it to the full. Eventually you'll be able to build up a sort of mental photo album of smells and associated memories.
Try ⇒ Task 55

HELP
The sense of smell, like all other senses, can be refined by practice. Just as a wine connoisseur can detect innumerable odours in a fine wine you will, with practice, be able to evoke memories simply by enlisting your sense of smell.

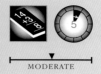

MODERATE

118 Clever Cuts

AIM This is an exercise that will test your visual imagination. It doesn't require any clever geometrical calculations, just a good eye.

TASK The figure below represents a ring (the centre is empty). Using only three straight cuts, see what is the greatest number of pieces you can make. You are not allowed to rearrange the pieces between cuts.

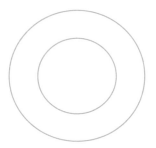

POOR
If you got far fewer than nine, you need to work on your visual skills. Try ➤ Task 62

AVERAGE
If you did this eventually, try pitting your wits against ➤ Task 84

BRILLIANT
If the answer to this one just leapt off the page at you, try ➤ Task 94

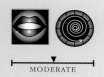

MODERATE

119 Town & Country

AIM The object of this game is to build vocabulary. If you think you're too grown up for this kind of thing, play it with your kids or shorten the time limit to something really challenging.

TASK Any number of people can play. First, write down a number of categories, for example, Town, Country, Song, Film, Book, Actor, Animal. You can have as many categories as you like. Then pick a letter at random (it's better to exclude X and Z for reasons that will become clear). Now you have three minutes to write down an entry in each category starting with the chosen letter. If you chose K the entries might be: Kirby, Kenya, Killing Me Softly, Karate Kid, Kidnapped, (Nicole) Kidman, Kinkajou. Alter the time limit to suit the abilities of the players.

POOR
If you're poor at this game you'll improve the more times you play it. Try ➤ Task 34

AVERAGE
The beauty of this game is that there is almost no limit to how much you can improve at it. Try ➤ Task 63

BRILLIANT
If you're that good you can help the other players to improve. In the meantime try ➤ Task 1

120 Flag Figure

AIM This is just a simple test of logic, but quite easy to get wrong.

TASK The Olympic flag bears five rings as shown:

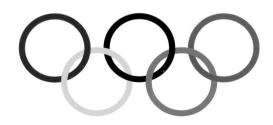

MODERATE

How many ways are there of arranging the five rings?

POOR
Anyone could work out such a puzzle given enough time, so the real challenge is to come up with a calculation that gives you the answer without a lot of counting. If you didn't get an answer at all, or took forever to work it out, you should have simply carried out the following calculation: 5 x 4 x 3 x 2 x 1.
Try ➤ Task **72**

AVERAGE
If you eventually worked this out the clever way, pat yourself on the back and try ➤ Task **84**

BRILLIANT
If this seemed transparently clear to you from the start then your powers of deduction are obviously in good order. Try ➤ Task **35**

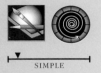

SIMPLE

121 Collage Creations

AIM For those who long to create something visual but are no good at drawing, this is a technique that might prove useful.

TASK Use pictures cut from magazines to make a collage like the one below. You can simply produce a pleasing picture or use your work to tell a story. To begin with this might seem a bit like something you did at primary school (because it is!), but you'll find that it is strangely soothing, thoroughly satisfying and addictive. The result needn't be a contender for the Turner Prize, as long as you use the process to access your creative ability.

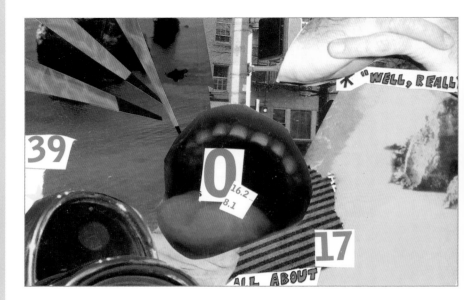

HELP
Anyone can do this. It only needs a bit of imagination and some time spent collecting the right images.

POOR
Oh, go on, you're just not trying! Try again. Keep swapping the pictures around until you get a result that says something to you. When you've had enough fun with this try
➤ Task **61**

AVERAGE
If you can produce something pleasing by this method – enjoy! Keep cutting out pictures and saving them for new collages. Old ones can always be adapted or simply torn down to make room for new efforts. Once you've had enough try
➤ Task **92**

BRILLIANT
If you really get a kick out of this, well done. Your only problem will be running out of walls to work on. Try ➤ Task **101**

122 Letter Pairs

MODERATE

AIM Is this really a word puzzle, a number puzzle or something quite different? The whole art of solving problems depends on recognizing what the problem is all about. Usually, once your mind is on the same wavelength as the person setting the puzzle, the answer is not that far away.

TASK Look at the following letter pairs. They all have something in common except for one. Which pair is the odd one out and why?

HR   AF   XS   MR   KF

POOR
If you didn't spot the answer you need more practice in how puzzles work.
Try ➤ Task 86

AVERAGE
If you got this but had to struggle a bit, try a different type of puzzle.
Try ➤ Task 15

BRILLIANT
If this was just too obvious for you, try something more challenging.
Try ➤ Task 12

Doing the task If the answer doesn't jump out and bite you, try writing out the alphabet and keeping it in front of you while doing the puzzle.

123 Magic Carpet

SIMPLE

AIM This is a form of relaxation guaranteed to produce a deep sleep and, very often, sweet dreams. It is useful for people suffering from stress.

TASK Start by lying on your bed. Make sure you are warm and comfortable and then carry out the Instant Relaxation exercise on page 97. Now that you are feeling calm, visualize your bed as a magic carpet and feel yourself floating in mid air. The carpet can hover or move at whatever speed you desire and go wherever you want. Now start the journey of your choice. You might want to gaze at a favourite piece of countryside from above, float over a sun-drenched beach or even travel the world. Of course, the carpet also functions in outer space, so a journey to the stars is no problem. You will find that you soon fall into a peaceful, happy sleep (and the carpet switches to autopilot as soon as you do so).

HELP
It is important when you begin this exercise to establish a few rules for yourself. The carpet is magic, so you cannot fall off or come to any harm whatsoever. Other air users (such as low flying jets) are not permitted anywhere near your airspace.

POOR
Go back to Basic Visualization and practise on something simple. When you have finished here try ➤ Task 32

AVERAGE
If you had limited success with this technique, keep trying because practice will make perfect.
Try ➤ Task 85

BRILLIANT
If this really helped you be sure to use all the other visualization techniques taught in this book.
Try ➤ Task 114

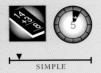

SIMPLE

124 Nines

AIM Here is a set of apparently random letters. How do you bring order to this confusion? Are they to be used as numbers, as parts of an anagram or do they have some other hidden significance? Once again, when you have unravelled the clue you should find the puzzle easy.

TASK Look carefully at the three-by-three letter grid. You will see that one of the letters is missing. There is a clue to help you: So to speak. When you discover what this is all about it should be obvious which letter you need to complete the grid.

E	R	A
P	T	N
S	E	?

POOR
If this one eluded you, try ➤ Task 89

AVERAGE
If you got this after some hard puzzling, try ➤ Task 90

BRILLIANT
Saw it straight away? Try something tougher in ➤ Task 104

Doing the task No ideas yet? Should you consider all the letters together, or are they broken up into vertical columns or horizontal rows? Think about that clue! It's really helpful when you get the right idea.

125 Body Clock

AIM As you know, your body has its own internal clock. Most of us wake up at the same times, eat at the same times and go to the bathroom at the same times every day. This internal rhythm is useful to us because it allows us to function without having to think about such mundane details each day. But the body clock can also be used as a memory aid, which is what the following exercise is all about.

TASK Take several days to examine the workings of your body clock. Make a careful note of the rhythm of your day. You'll find that not only do you do things like eating and sleeping at regular times, but that your mood changes according to the time of day. When you have a thorough understanding of biorhythms you can start to associate other activities with these. For example, when you get the urge to drink coffee after you arrive at work, you can associate this with remembering to check your diary. When you start to feel hungry in the late morning use it as a signal to make some important phone calls. You can't use this technique to remind you of lists of information, but it is a good regular reminder of routine chores that need to be done.

POOR
If this one didn't prove a hit for you it doesn't matter. Maybe your body clock doesn't tick as regularly as some.
Try ➤ Task 47

AVERAGE
Try ➤ Task 27

BRILLIANT
Try ➤ Task 55

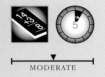

MODERATE

126 Prized Possession?

AIM Lateral-thinking puzzles work by giving you incomplete or misleading information. To solve the puzzle you need to read the wording very carefully and then look for the holes in what it tells you. This one overlooks one very basic fact. As soon as you know what that is, the answer becomes obvious.

TASK You buy it, though you don't really want one. If you can't afford to buy it, you get given one. It protects you even though you don't need protection. It often continues working long after it's been disposed of. What is it?

HELP
Why would you buy it if you didn't want it? In what unusual circumstance might you buy something to protect you even if you didn't need protecting? How is it disposed of?

POOR	AVERAGE	BRILLIANT
If you didn't get it your thinking was not flexible enough. Try ➡ Task 50	**If you got this – even after long cogitation – well done!** Try ➡ Task 40	**Was it just too easy for you?** Try ➡ Task 90

MODERATE

127 Four Square

AIM This is a test of logical thinking. It requires only primary maths but, even so, will prove tricky for some.

TASK Look at the four squares. What letter should go in the centre of the square on the right?

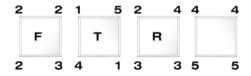

HELP
There is no clever way to do this, though there are many stupid ones. The trick is to discover the simple formula that governs all the squares.

POOR	AVERAGE	BRILLIANT
Haven't got a clue? If you've worked out that the letters are really thinly disguised numbers, then all you need to do is work out the formula. Try ➡ Task 91	**If you got this you can be pleased with yourself. It's amazing how difficult a simple calculation becomes once the rules are made obscure.** Try ➡ Task 94	**If you cut through this with the samurai sword of your logic you are a person to be feared.** Try ➡ Task 105

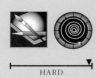

128 Cut!

AIM Before you accuse me of going to extremes I should point out that what follows is a genuine creative writing technique that has been used effectively by several famous modern writers.

TASK It is very difficult sometimes to get enough spontaneity into your writing. Too often you look back at what you wrote and see pages of dull, flat prose. A number of writers (mainly American) tried the following. When you have finished writing, take your work and cut each page into quarters, or even eighths. Then mix all the pieces up, put them back into pages and read the whole thing through again. Too crazy? Couldn't possibly work? If you're really into extreme experiences you'll retype it just as it is and let your readers make of it what they will. If, however, you are not quite that avant-garde you can use the mixed-up version as the basis for a new attempt which, with luck, will gain in spontaneity from the mixing process.

POOR
If you didn't get anything out of this but a nasty mess, ask yourself why? Perhaps you're still not willing to let yourself go.
Try ❱ Task 6

AVERAGE
If you see possibilities in this then try to take it further. The element of chaos will help loosen up your writing and make way for exciting discoveries.
Try ❱ Task 32

BRILLIANT
If you enjoyed this and found that it worked well for you try ❱ Task 8

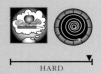

HARD

129 Symbols

AIM The aim of this task is to memorize the table below. It is intentionally difficult (you may not even know the names of some of letters and symbols involved).

TASK Study the table below for as long as you wish. The aim of this test is accuracy rather than speed. Even if some of the symbols are unfamiliar you should be able to learn to reproduce them well enough to be recognizable. You may use whatever method of study you prefer (my preference would be to study one column at a time from left to right). Test yourself as you go. You might think that you remember but, unless you can reproduce the table without looking at the original, you'll never be certain that you have it stored in your memory.

$	Z	¥	Õ	∂
&	μ	®	Δ	Ω
§	#	¢	ß	Σ
Ø	Æ	Ñ	√	Ç
±	@	£	≥	π

HELP
Make up names of your own for the symbols you don't know, for example, you can call § a double S.

POOR
If you found this difficult, don't be surprised. It is difficult. If, after about 30 minutes, you still can't do it, then move try
» Task 14

AVERAGE
If you have the whole thing off by heart in 10–15 minutes you've done well.
Try » Task 73

BRILLIANT
If you could do this perfectly in less than 10 minutes your recall is excellent. See if you still remember it in a week's time. For the moment try
» Task 87

130 Day Disorder

AIM This is purely an exercise in clear thinking. The problem is actually quite easy but the wording makes your brain ache.

TASK When the day before yesterday was referred to as 'the day after tomorrow', the day that was then called 'yesterday' was as far away from the day we now call 'tomorrow' as yesterday is from the day on which we shall now be able to speak of last Monday as 'a week ago yesterday'. What day is it?

POOR	AVERAGE	BRILLIANT
Yes, you can do it, although it may feel as if you can't. The trick is to clarify all the bits that have been inserted to bamboozle you. Try ⟫ Task 64	If you solved this in the time allowed that's pretty good. If you did it without having to write anything down that's even better. Try ⟫ Task 82	If you're the sort of person who can see straight through all the verbiage and get the answer immediately, then congratulations. Try ⟫ Task 91

SIMPLE

HELP
If you have trouble doing this in your head try drawing a time line.

131 Circle Story

AIM This is a creative exercise for several people – four to six would be perfect. Its aim is to get them to work in co-operation to produce a coherent story.

TASK The group should sit in a circle. Decide between you how long each speaker's turn is to last and who is going to start. You can, if you wish, decide in advance what the theme of your story will be. Record each session for later examination. There are two ways to play the game. One is the party version where you all work to build a wild, fantastical and, probably, nonsensical narrative. Or you can play a serious version where you try seriously to outline the plot of a 'real' story. Both versions have their good points.

POOR	AVERAGE	BRILLIANT
If the experiment doesn't work you could try changing the setting to make people feel more relaxed. If that doesn't help, look at the group and consider why they are not working well together. Try ⟫ Task 16	If you get something of a story out of this, keep going and try to improve your output. Let people take a turn the moment they feel they have something important to contribute. Try ⟫ Task 29	If you get a good plot this way, the next step is to work on fleshing it out. You can do this individually or collectively. If you work individually you'll have fun seeing the number of directions your original plot took. Try ⟫ Task 32

HARD

HELP
This can work superbly well or be an embarrassment, depending on the people involved. It is important to work in a group where the members feel comfortable with each other. Creativity of this sort is a little like taking off your clothes – you have to show people a part of yourself that is usually private. If you don't have confidence in your colleagues it just won't work.

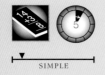

SIMPLE

132 Letter Logic 2

AIM This puzzle is really simple, but only once you realize what it's all about. Until then it's just a jumble of letters! Is it verbal or numerical? Is it about the shapes of the letters or is there some lateral thinking involved? Think hard.

TASK All you have to do is look at the two rows of letters and supply a third row of your own. Once you are on the right track you'll soon realize it because the answer is a six-letter word.

L	P	U	J	Z	Y
G	B	L	C	M	X
?	?	?	?	?	?

POOR
If you didn't crack this one your problem is probably just that you didn't work out what the puzzle was all about. Success in solving puzzles depends not so much on great brainpower as on keeping your mind alert to all the possibilities. Try ➤ Task 61

AVERAGE
If you did this one but needed all the time allowed, then go to ➤ Task 24 to see if you can crack it more quickly.

BRILLIANT
If you weren't fooled for a moment, try something a bit harder in ➤ Task 36

Doing the task If the method of solving this isn't obvious, write the alphabet down and pick out the pairs of letters. A pattern will emerge.

133 Around The House

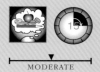

AIM This is a memory technique that uses visualization. It is useful for remembering a limited amount of information in the short term.

TASK For this exercise you need to see a familiar place, such as your own house, in your mind's eye. Let's say that you need to remember a list of things to do. First you must divide your list into sections, such as things to do at home, at work and social arrangements, and so on. Assign one room of the house to each section. Now, mentally, go into each room and leave yourself a note about each task in a separate place. If you can make the place appropriate to the task, so much the better. For example, if you need to buy your wife an anniversary present, mentally leave a note in her place at the dining table. If you need to complete a report for your boss, leave a note lying on the desk in your study. When you want to recall the information, just visit the appropriate room and pick up the notes.

POOR
If your visual imagination is poor, don't bother to try the more complicated version of this technique, but go straight to ➤ Task 14

AVERAGE
As with all visualizations, the more often you use it the more powerful it becomes. If you have moderate success with this technique then keep trying. Try ➤ Task 10

BRILLIANT
If this sort of visualization comes easily to you, go to Memory Lane in ➤ Task 96 for a more advanced version of the technique.

HELP
When you have used the technique you must remember to go around and empty all the locations you no longer need so that they can be used again. You can, of course, always add more locations as the need arises.

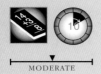

MODERATE

134 Dodgy Digits

AIM Here's a test of your numerical reasoning. It should keep you occupied for a little while.

TASK In this puzzle the ten digits of zero to nine are each represented by the letters of a 10-letter word in which no letters are repeated. NIGHTMARES would be an example though, of course, not the correct word. Use the following addition sum to work out what the word is:

$$\begin{array}{ccccc} G & A & U & N & T \\ O & I & L & E & R \\ \hline R & G & U & O & E & I \end{array}$$

POOR	**AVERAGE**	**BRILLIANT**
If you found this too hard then figures may not be your thing. Even so, have another try by going to ➤ Task **80**	If you got this (even in extra time), you did well. Try ➤ Task **127**	For someone with a head for figures this question should be simple. You, presumably, are such a person. Try ➤ Task **105**

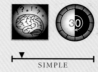

135 Rhymes

AIM Rhyming is a very powerful memory aid. The task of this section is to learn how to use it effectively.

TASK Strictly speaking the technique relies on metre more than on rhyme, though where you can make a rhyme it is an added bonus. Be careful how you use this technique! It is a very strong memory glue that will fix things in your mind for a long time and maybe even forever.

Just for fun let's learn the Presidents of the USA. The first four are easy because they have a natural rhythm. Try saying without Washington, Adams, Jefferson, Madison without introducing a metre – it's almost impossible! The rest will provide more of a challenge:

Washington, Adams, Jefferson, Madison,

Monroe and Adams, Jackson, Van Buren,

Harrison, Tyler, Knox Polk and Taylor,

Fillmore and Pierce, Buchanan and Lincoln,

Johnson and Grant, Hayes and Garfield,

Arthur and Cleveland, Harrison, Cleveland,

McKinley, Roosevelt, Taft and Wilson,

Harding and Coolidge, Hoover and Roosevelt,

Truman and Eisenhower, Kennedy, Johnson,

Nixon and Ford, Carter and Reagan.

George Bush and Bill Clinton,

And George W. Bush.

OK, now try learning it a couple of lines at a time. Use a really sing-song voice just the way you were taught not to read poetry at school. In half an hour you should have the whole thing. Come back to the task a couple of times over the next few days and again in a couple of weeks' time. You'll find you can do the whole list without a slip.

POOR	AVERAGE	BRILLIANT
If you can't do this at first, keep trying. The more pronounced the rhythm you use the better it will work. Try ❯❯ Task 79	If you can do this you can use the same technique for other things. A non-scanning rhythm may be more memorable. Try ❯❯ Task 98	If this really worked for you, then add it to your memory toolbox and use it whenever you need to fix information. Now try ❯❯ Task 77

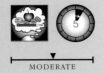

MODERATE

136 A Flash Of Inspiration

AIM Sometimes the old methods are the best. Here is a reminder of the flashcards you probably used as a kid at school. Childish, undoubtedly, but very effective. Don't be proud!

TASK Photocopy the page opposite and cut out the flashcards. Look at the Chinese characters and see if you can memorize their meanings in less than five minutes. Come back to the exercise tomorrow and see whether you can still remember them. The characters given have been chosen for particular reasons.

HELP
Think of the characters as pictures (which, indeed, some of them are). The dots around the heart represent beats, the ear is purely pictorial, as are the mountain and the sun. The character for gold represents a forge (see the roof at the top?). That just leaves melon to remember.

POOR
Found it difficult? Maybe Chinese is not your thing. You would need to memorize thousands of characters far more complicated than these to be able to read a newspaper.
Try ▶ Task 14

AVERAGE
If you found this useful you should consider adapting the technique for use in other contexts.
Try ▶ Task 27

BRILLIANT
If you found this easy, then add the technique to your collection of memory tools.
Try ▶ Task 55

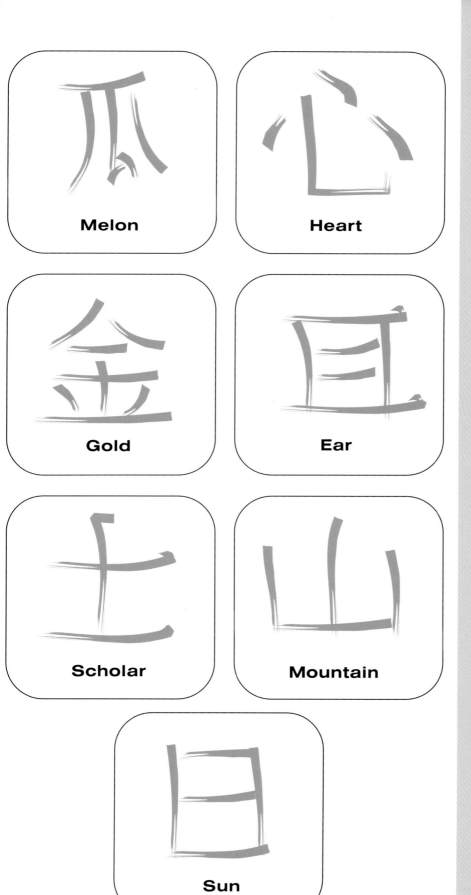

Melon

Heart

Gold

Ear

Scholar

Mountain

Sun

Answers

2 Parts Problem C (12), E (14).

4 Misfit DANDELION is the only one not used as a girl's name.

7 Boudicca's Birthday There were 129 years between the birth of Cleopatra and the death of Boudicca but, as their combined ages came to only 100 years, there must have been 29 years between their lives. Therefore Boudicca must have been born 29 years after the death of Cleopatra in 30 BC. This makes the date of her birth 1 BC.

9 Letter Logic SWIMWEAR.

12 Dear Departed Two widows each had a son, and each widow married the son of the other and had a daughter by the marriage.

15 Triangle Trouble The letters spell JOHN F KENNEDY. The F is missing.

19 Princess Yasmin's Maze Only number three can reach Yasmin's chamber.

21 Picking Pairs

Line 1	7
Line 2	8
Line 3	8
Line 4	9
Line 5	7
Total	39

22 Sentence Search Patriotism is not enough.

23 Ball Bother They pee in the hole. Yes, the answer is gross and that may have been what put off of you thinking of it. You were told at the outset to consider every possibility.

25 Sarah's Game

S	A	H	A	H	A	R	S	A	R
A	S	A	R	H	R	A	H	A	S
R	A	S	R	S	S	H	A	S	R
H	A	S	R	S	A	H	A	R	A
A	S	A	H	R	A	R	A	A	S
S	H	A	R	A	S	A	R	A	R
A	S	A	R	H	R	S	A	H	A
R	A	H	S	A	S	R	A	H	A
A	S	A	R	R	H	H	S	A	S
H	A	R	A	H	A	S	A	R	A

26 Crossed Uncrossed The whole game hinges on whether the player passing the object has their legs crossed when making the pass.

27 Lunch Bunch 1. Six, 2. Lasagne, 3. Angela, 4. Two, 5. Jenny, 6. John, 7. Graham, 8. Jenny, 9. Fajita, 10, Craig.

28 Word Wheel MATTE, INGLE, SLAVE, THESE, LOUSE, EAGLE, TRIPE, ORATE, EVADE. The initials form the word MISTLETOE.

29 Candide Caper Time

30 Will he Win? The money was given to the charity, which then wrote Augustus a cheque for the entire sum. The cheque was buried with him.

33 Box Clever You can make two boxes (A and E).

35 What's in a Name? They are all anagrams of girls' names.

36 Cross Quiz Ben's age is 10 16/21 years, John's is 29 15/21, and Kate's is 24 20/21

40 Fifteen Squared

2	9	4
7	5	3
6	1	8

44 Small change

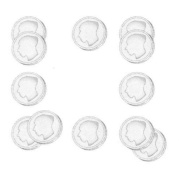

46 Code breaker 1 Secret Code:

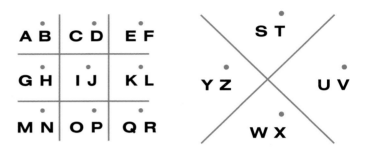

48 Colour Conundrum White.

51 Same Difference They all have a past tense that rhymes with 'fort'.

50 Trump trick

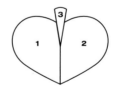 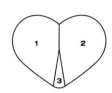

53 What Next?

The letters are the second letter of the days of the week (Monday, Tuesday, Wednesday, Thursday, Friday, Saturday, Sunday.)

56 Pizza Poser They were grandmother, mother and daughter. They cut the pizza into six and had two pieces each.

58 Cubist conundrum

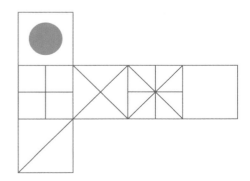

60 Memory Mall

1. Carpet Heaven (1970)
2. Blossoms
3. Carpet Heaven
4. A Piece of Cake
5. Man About Town
6. Curls
7. Fish (from Dave's Plaice next door)
8. Sparks
9. Mike's Bikes
10. Blossoms and Curls

61 A Third Way 5832, 17496

68 Bermuda triangle 11. Add all the outer numbers together and place the sum in the centre.

69 Second thoughts The all look the same when viewed upside down on a calculator.

72 Code breaker 3 Give Peace a Chance.

78 Maze murder

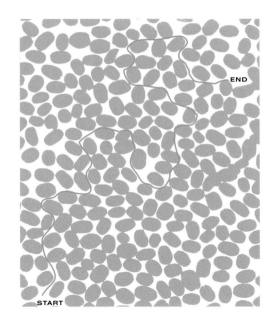

80 They are the seconds on a defective digital clock.

84 The skyscraper was 85 floors high. When the man hit the ground he died, of course.

86 Frustrating Figures

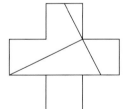 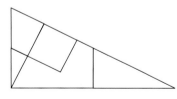 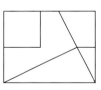

88 Match mystery Place three matches flat on the table and use the others to make a pyramid.

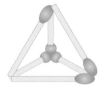

90 Lightfoot TERPSICHOREAN

91 Star Strategy BLACK, STAIN, BRAVE, STAVE, BRAIN. You can also make out the name STALIN.

94 Clock Conundrum

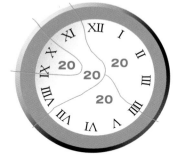

97 Wonky Words
Y, giving FAIRLY, FAMILY, RATIFY, SHAGGY, GRASSY, TRASHY.

98 Alphabet Soup Line 1: 6 pairs, Line 2: 6 pairs, Line 3: 7 pairs

99 Penny Lane

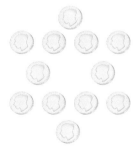

100 Similar Circles D. It is the only one that is symmetrical.

102 Cola Conundrum Drink until the level of liquid runs from the lip of the glass to the top of the opposite bottom rim. There will then be exactly half left

104 Three By Three 6. The numbers in each grid add up to 47.

105 Name Game O. The letters form the word EPONYMOUS in a simple substitution code in which A = W, B = X, C = Y, D = Z, E = A, etc.

107 Code Breaker 2 We wish you a Merry Christmas. The grid contains all the letters of the alphabet (I and J double up). Co-ordinates are provided by the letters A–E running down the side of the grid and numerals 1–5 along the top.

108 Horseshoe Conundrum
Make cut AB. Then put the pieces together so that you can cut CD, EF and GH all at one snip.

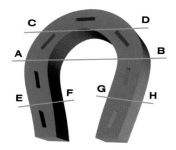

111 Shapely Problem The circle.

113 Cubic Challenge 12/64

116 Delinquent Driver There were five people in the men's car, the driver being a woman.

118 Clever Cuts You can make 9 pieces.

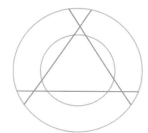

120 Flag Figure 120.

122 Letter Pairs HR. The others are all equally far apart from each other in the alphabet.

124 Nines ANSWER The letters make the word ESPERANTO (the artificial international language).

126 Prized Possession? The question leads you to consider decisions that a living person would make. It leads you away from the idea that the subject of the puzzle is dead. Of course, the answer is a coffin.

127 Four Square Y. Bottom left x bottom right x top right divided by top left = number of letter in alphabetical order.

130 Day Disorder Thursday.

132 Letter Logic The puzzle depends on alphanumeric values. Each letter is worth a number based on its position in the alphabet (so A = 1, B= 2, C= 3, and so on). Subtract the bottom row from the top, then turn the resulting numbers back into letters, and you get the word ENIGMA.

134 Dodgy Digits The word is REGULATION.

Index
References given are task numbers not page numbers

Author's Acknowledgement

With many thanks to my daughter, Gina, who provided much of the original artwork. I'd also like to thank my late friend Harold Gale who taught me how to write puzzles, thereby ensuring I had an income for life. Finally, I'd like to acknowledge Henry Dudeney, one of the greatest puzzle writers of all time, some of whose classic conundrums I have borrowed.